APPLES
AND
PEARS

APPLES AND PEARS

A revolutionary diet programme for
weight loss and optimum health

Dr MARIE SAVARD

with Carol Svec

Vermilion
LONDON

1 3 5 7 9 10 8 6 4 2

Copyright © Dr Marie Savard 2005

Dr Marie Savard has asserted her moral right to be identified as the author of this work in accordance with the Copyright, Design and Patents Act 1988.

First published in the United States in 2005 by Atria Books, Simon & Schuster, Inc.

First published in the United Kingdom in 2005 by
Vermilion, an imprint of Ebury Publishing
Random House UK Ltd.
Random House
20 Vauxhall Bridge Road
London SW1V 2SA

Random House Australia (Pty) Limited
20 Alfred Street, Milsons Point, Sydney,
New South Wales 2061, Australia

Random House New Zealand Limited
18 Poland Road, Glenfield,
Auckland 10, New Zealand

Random House (Pty) Limited
Endulini, 5A Jubilee Road, Parktown 2193, South Africa

Random House UK Limited Reg. No. 954009

www.randomhouse.co.uk

Papers used by Vermilion are natural, recyclable products made from wood grown in sustainable forests.

Exercise photographs used with permission and copyrighted by The Hygenic Corporation, 2004

Designed by Jaime Putorti

A CIP catalogue record is available for this book from the British Library.

ISBN 0 09 190646 6

Printed and bound in Great Britain by
Clays Ltd, St Ives plc

For Brad, Zach, Aaron and Ben –
you are simply the best!

Acknowledgements

I have dedicated my entire career to empowering women to take charge of their health and to work in collaborative partnerships with their health practitioners. Women make most of the health care decisions for their families, yet too often they leave for last the most important person in their lives – themselves! First and foremost I dedicate this book to all women, including the thousands of women I have cared for or interacted with over the years. I hope this book will provide the information and inspiration that every woman needs to be as healthy as possible.

I need to thank the most important men in my life – my husband, Bradley Fenton, and our three sons, Zachary, Aaron and Ben. They have always been my greatest source of purpose, inspiration and support. For years they have listened to my frustrations about a broken health care system that fails to put people at the centre of their care, and now they listen with interest to my observations about women and the powerful role body shape plays in forecasting one's health destiny.

My parents have always been there for me, eagerly supporting every project I have undertaken – reading drafts of my work and offering their wise perspective. A special thanks to my mom for sharing with me her experience as a participant in America's famous Nurses' Health Study, which has been the source of so much important information for women. Eileen is one of the best sisters anyone could have. She has stood by me as a colleague and friend ever since I began talking about patient empowerment and provided the graphic design assistance that helped make the *Apples & Pears* concept come alive. My sister Millie's story was the source of much of my passion and drive to get the life-saving information about body shape to as many women as possible so that they can take the steps they need to take before it is too late. My five other brothers and sisters have helped me in more ways than they realize, as well.

My agent and former editor, Jessica Papin of Dystel & Goderich Literary Management, believed in the purpose of my work and my ability to take my message to a larger audience from the very beginning, long before I realized this myself. Thank you. And thanks also to Jane Dystel, who had the insight and wisdom to suggest Carol Svec as a writing partner.

I also thank my colleagues at Atria Books, who welcomed me with an excitement and enthusiasm far greater than I could have ever imagined. Brenda Copeland, our editor, recognised the significance of this book and that women's health care could be transformed as a result.

For the photographs in this book, I would like to thank Philip Savard, as well as the Thera-Band company. Special thanks, too, to Tara Smith, R.D., who provided nutrition guidance; Jill Kleinberg, P.T., M.H.A., who provided exercise guidance; and Mark Anderson and the dedicated staff at Thera-Band for their technical assistance. I owe a multitude of thanks to the women who volunteered to have their pictures taken and shared with the world – you prove that all women are beautiful. These include Sharon Ayscue, Shannon Louise Childs, Pamela Conner, Stephanie Conner, Judy Corderman, Karen DeBord, Pam Etu, Theresa M. Ferree, Carnela Hill, Sheena Cain Johnson, Joanna Jones, Jill Kleinberg, Eileen Mackison, Tammy McWilliams, Rhonda Nelson, Diane Resh, Angie Savard, Nannette Smith, Denise Stottlemyer, Stephanie Stump, Rhonda Sutton, Susan Upadhyay, Rose Welt and Hong Zhou.

Carol Svec also thanks Ann Agrawal, Asha Agrawal, Teresa Lawrence, Marina and Ted Rudisill, Joanna and Alan Jones, and Rhonda Sutton, who read and commented on early drafts; Peter Guzzardi, for moral support and spinach salad; Sid Kirchheimer for the usual reasons; and Megan Lawrence, the photographer's assistant, who never gets enough credit. Thanks also to Bob and Sharon Hill, the thoughtful hosts of the 'Round House' in Duck, North Carolina, for sharing their little piece of paradise. And a special note of gratitude for Bill Svec for being a tireless source of inspiration and humour.

Finally, I would like to thank Carol Svec, my writing colleague, who not only listened and understood my message immediately but became an instant friend and collaborator. Together we accomplished so much more than I could have on my own. (Carol says, *Ditto, Marie!*)

Contents

Introduction

Show me a woman – any woman – and I can forecast her health destiny just by observing her body shape. I know who will probably die of heart disease or breast cancer, who will have a rough transition through menopause, who will likely end up with a broken hip and who may not live long enough to celebrate her 70th birthday. I am rarely wrong. From my 30 years of clinical experience and a review of decades of research, I've discovered that *the single most powerful predictor of a woman's future health is the shape of her body.*

All women's bodies can be categorised as either 'apple-shaped' or 'pear-shaped', depending on where they are most likely to put on fat, even if they aren't currently overweight. Women who tend to gain weight around their waists are said to have apple-shaped bodies because, like the fruit, their weight collects around their middles. Women who tend to add extra pounds around their hips, buttocks and thighs are said to have pear-shaped bodies because, like the fruit, they are widest at the bottom. These terms have been around for decades, but they have mainly been used as physical descriptions, much the way we might say that a woman is blonde or brunette. Only now are we realising the powerful physiologic effects of being either an 'apple' or a 'pear'.

Body shape is not something we get to choose; we have very little control over our basic underlying proportions. Contrary to popular belief, people don't develop a pear shape simply because they sit on their bottoms most of the time. The human body is not a loose bag of sand in which the weight goes to our lowest point. If that were true, our feet would be the size of watermelons. These two shape categories are fundamental, genetically influenced patterns that affect much more than how we look in a bikini. Body shape is related to differences in our physical chemistry, hormone production and sensitivity, metabolism, and possibly even personality. Have you tried the latest fad diet but found you still couldn't lose weight while everyone else managed to drop two trouser sizes? Chances are that that particular diet wasn't right for your body shape. Ever wonder why some women suffer through intolerable hot flushes during menopause while others sail right through? Or why hormone therapy makes some women feel healthy and happy, while making other women feel bloated and irritable? Again, blame it on body shape. Our shape affects our likelihood of developing heart disease, osteoporosis, the metabolic syndrome, diabetes, stroke, varicose veins, breast cancer and endometrial cancer. Body shape also gives clues to which adolescent girls are more likely to develop eating disorders, which types of exercise are best, and which emotions can physically change our shape. It even tells us our chances for living to be old enough to have to worry about nursing home care.

Physicians and researchers have been talking about the importance of body shape for years, but this health message has not been fully explained to the people who can use it most – women in general. The scientific information in *Apples and Pears* has never before been analysed and collected in a single consumer publication, so what you are reading now is the cutting edge of women's health information. In the coming chapters, you will learn how and why different body shapes benefit from customised diets, exercise regimens, medications, menopause therapies, psychosocial interventions and lifestyle changes. Women who follow the action items for better health will be able to transcend their biology to lose weight, increase energy and decrease their risks for type 2 diabetes, heart disease, breast cancer and osteoporosis. In short, I'm going to tell you everything I know about how you can look great and feel wonderful, regardless of your current weight or body shape.

Putting all the pieces of the body shape puzzle together was one of those 'Aha!' moments for me. It began decades ago when I watched my mother dutifully complete lengthy surveys that were sent to her every few years. She would have to detail her every health move, including what she ate, how much exercise she did, what she weighed, which medical conditions she had and which medications she was taking. My father remembers searching the house for a flexible tape measure to help my mother record her waist size. (This turned out to be a tough task – my dad was an engineer and carpenter and only had metal or wooden rulers.) What could they possibly want with that information? he asked himself. Now we know. You see, my mother is part of the now-famous Nurses' Health Study, which has been recording the lifestyle choices and medical conditions of more than 120,000 women nurses since 1976. Much of what we know and teach about women's health today comes from this ongoing study, and from subsequent studies of younger nurses and their daughters.

A summary of the findings from that study was published in 2001 in a wonderful book titled *Healthy Women, Healthy Lives,* which my mother gave to me as a gift. (She knew that I would be proud of her contribution to this landmark study, especially because I had been a nurse before becoming a physician and had a special interest in women's health.) As I read through the book, I noticed that the concept of body shape was an ever-present, although not central, observation with regard to disease risk. What kept jumping off the page for me were all the references to apple-shaped women – and their higher risks of developing heart disease, type 2 diabetes, stroke and breast cancer.

Aha! I already understood to some degree the importance of body shape in predicting the risk of heart disease. I knew, for example, that men and women who carry most of their body fat around their middles have a much higher risk of having a heart attack than pear-shaped people. But I didn't understand the profound impact that shape could have on risk for a host of conditions – including cancer, osteoporosis (the bone-thinning disease of old age), varicose veins and even eating disorders – until I started looking at the medical literature. Then I found evidence everywhere. It was overwhelming. When it comes to overall health, body shape really does matter!

MY FAMILY'S MIXED BASKET

Of course, I really only needed to look within my own family to see what I had missed all along. I am one of eight children (I have three brothers and four sisters). Most of us girls have subtle variations of the pear shape – we always tended to have 'small tops and big bottoms'. For as long as I can remember, whenever I shopped for new clothes, I always tried on the trousers of a suit first because my bottom was the hardest part to fit. To this day I prefer to wear trousers to cover my larger-than-I-like legs, instead of the short skirts that many apple-shaped women (with their typically beautiful legs) can wear.

Three of my four sisters had similar concerns. My fourth sister, Millie, had a much different experience, and a more serious problem. Unlike my other sisters, Millie has an apple-shaped body. True to her type, she has great legs, which always made the rest of us a little envious. But over the years, she has gained weight primarily around her middle. Although she must have had an apple shape her whole life, I didn't really notice until later in life when her midsection became more rounded and she lost whatever waist she had in her youth. Millie now has a number of serious medical conditions, including type 2 diabetes, high blood pressure, abnormally high blood fats in a worrisome pattern and osteoarthritis of her knees. Her diabetes has led to other complications, including nerve damage (neuropathy) in her feet, causing constant burning and pain. For years Millie had been told about her borderline blood sugar levels, but she was never told how something as innocent-sounding as 'blood sugar' could devastate her body. Nor was she ever told that it was within her power to avoid serious disease. In fact, Millie recently requested her old medical records from a previous physician and discovered that she had had borderline blood glucose readings for many, many years, but her doctor had never told her. After years of ignorance, she was ultimately diagnosed and treated for diabetes.

Today, Millie manages her blood sugar, blood pressure and blood fats with a combination of medications and major lifestyle changes. Even the pain of her neuropathy is better now that she is controlling her diabetes. But if only she could turn back the clock, she could have avoided many of the health problems that plague her now. Millie was born to be apple-shaped. Throughout her adolescence, into adulthood, and past menopause, her body followed a pattern that made her more likely to develop particular diseases. If we had known then what we know now, she could have prevented much of the damage that has already been done. That's what this book is all about – recognising the risk, then taking action to stop the process of disease and decline.

My mother has a different story. My mother had the classic pear shape, or hourglass shape, that was once revered. After she passed through menopause, however, her body began to change. My mother was too busy raising and worrying about her eight children to take the time to care for herself. She rarely went to the doctor, never monitored her health, and slowly gained weight. Like many pear-shaped women who were used to finding inches added to their hips and thighs, my mother didn't notice the redistribution of fat and creeping weight gain around her waist. Eventually, my mother's shape shifted from pear to apple. At age 65, my mother suffered a massive heart attack. Suddenly her health was in the spotlight for the first time in decades. She learned that the physical changes that occurred with menopause and ageing led to a big increase in her blood pressure and blood cholesterol, and she had become a walking time bomb for heart attack.

My sister Millie and my mother represent two ends of the spectrum of apple-shaped women. You can be born with a genetic predisposition to be apple-shaped, as Millie was (my father's side has a history of diabetes and I suspect they were apple-shaped); or you can gradually become apple-shaped after menopause, as my mother did.

My passion to write this book comes from these family stories and the stories of countless other women I have cared for and treated over the years. It is with the clarity of hindsight that I see that I could have made an even bigger difference in my patients' health if only I had recognised sooner the diagnostic importance of body shape. But back then, I didn't have the *language of body shape* to begin the conversation. It is difficult to take the first step to speak up and interfere with someone else's health choices; talking about body shape would have provided an easy transition into a discussion of weight, lifestyle and disease risk. I could have told them that, through no fault of their own, body shape had put their health in danger. The good news is that we know now. And there are things we can do to prevent or even reverse the disease process set in motion by 'appleness'.

Pear-shaped women have their own set of problems. In our image-conscious society, fat thighs and large buttocks are mocked. Even gorgeous, pear-shaped Jennifer Lopez has had to endure years of negative commentary about her figure. There's the joke that may or may not have originated on *Late Night with Conan O'Brien,* but which has circulated on the internet: when Jennifer Lopez got a massage, Sean Puffy Combs came in with her and told the massage therapist not to touch her rear end. The massage therapist said he wouldn't have been able to massage Jennifer Lopez's rear end anyway because she only booked a half day. Frances O'Toole, in *The Observer,* contributed her own take on J-Lo's figure: 'This isn't a catwalk bottom – it may be firm, but it's covered in fat.' These are the messages that contribute to women being unable to accept themselves. Pear-shaped women who internalise the rail-thin ideal of fashion models end up struggling with body image problems throughout their lives. It's no wonder that they suffer from eating disorders more often than apple-shaped women do. What they don't know is that losing weight will not change the overall shape of their bodies – it will only make them smaller pears. After menopause, pear-shaped women are more likely than apple-shaped women to develop osteoporosis. And like my mother, pear-shaped women can become apple-shaped, increasing their risk for disease while adding inches to their waists. For these women, this book outlines how to sidestep the physical and emotional pitfalls of being a pear, and what can be done to avoid turning into an apple.

The overall purpose of this book is to change the way women and their physicians perceive their bodies and understand their disease risk. I have made it my life's mission to empower every woman to take charge of her health. When the woman is my patient, I can sit her down, explain the importance of body shape in the context of her family history, current medical conditions and lifestyle and warn her of her specific disease risks. Then, with medical recommendations customised by body shape, I can tell her exactly what she needs to do in order to *live longer, lose weight and feel healthier*. For the millions of other women in the world, the ones I can't treat personally, I am putting that same power in their hands with *Apples and Pears*.

This book is divided into three parts. Part 1 discusses body shape in general – the differences between body shapes, how to determine your shape, the different kinds of fat and its distribution patterns, and how different life stages can affect weight and shape. These chapters provide the framework for understanding and interpreting the information in the rest of the book.

Part 2 provides in-depth information about medical issues, including the body shape connection to the metabolic syndrome, type 2 diabetes, inflammation, heart disease, cancer, osteoporosis, varicose veins, stress and depression. The chapter on hormones provides answers about birth control pills and hormone therapy – who might benefit and who should avoid them entirely.

Part 3 provides customised diet recommendations for apple-shaped women and pear-shaped women, as well as the most effective ways to lose weight and the most promising exercises. Plus, I provide a Body Shape Health Log blank for you to copy and use to track your health and weight loss progress.

By the end of this book, you will understand the health risks faced by women with your body shape. You'll be able to identify your particular weak points, and you'll know how to make them stronger. You'll be able to talk with your doctor about how to incorporate body shape into your wellness plan, and you'll be more confident in the health decisions you make. In addition, you will have a whole new way to think about your body – not as an enemy to be punished and hated, but as a dynamic reflection of your genetic and personal history. I've been told by women time and again that once they understood the concepts in this book, they were finally able to feel happy in their own skin. That's how powerful the concept of body shape is; it can affect both our health and our happiness. The mission of this book is to help you learn to harness that power for yourself.

The *Apples and Pears* Promise

No matter how many diets or exercise regimens have failed you in the past, no matter what your current weight is or how long you've gone without taking care of yourself, no matter if you are a teenager just becoming aware of body shape or a woman who has gone through menopause and is facing new health challenges, this book will change the way you relate to your body forever. You will start to see yourself and your friends differently, in a more accepting manner. You may even learn to love the body you've been fighting against your whole life. You will discover simple things you can do to become thinner, healthier, stronger, and more in control of your medical destiny. Of course, the actions you take are up to you, but the knowledge alone is power. I'm hoping this book will be your 'Aha!' moment.

PART ONE

ABOUT BODY SHAPE

CHAPTER I

Apples and Pears

Body shape is the closest thing we have to a medical crystal ball. This one simple piece of information is more important than weight for predicting your risk of heart disease or stroke. It can foretell your likelihood of developing type 2 diabetes 10 to 20 years before blood tests show a problem with blood sugar, and it is as powerful as family history for revealing a tendency towards breast cancer, endometrial cancer or osteoporosis. The good news is that this crystal ball only shows what is *likely* to happen; our health destiny is not written in stone. We have the power to improve the course of our lives in spite of our shapes . . . *if* we are willing to take action.

But body shape tells us much more than our risk of future disease. Want to understand the reasons for your cellulite, bloated belly, depression, low self-esteem, menopausal hot flushes, gestational diabetes or varicose veins? In many cases, everything you need to know can be found in the measurements of your waist, hips and buttocks. Ever wonder why exercise never slims your 'thunder thighs', or why you gain weight when you're under stress, or why diets never seem to work for you? Again, body shape reveals all.

Once you understand what body shape means, how it is formed, how it changes and how it relates to your health, the effect is like ripping off a blindfold. *Finally* your stomach and thighs make sense. *Finally* you know what you have to do to lose weight more easily. *Finally* you can put medical problems in context and really know what to do to improve them. *Finally* you can appreciate and understand your body as it is, while still nurturing it to become stronger and healthier than ever before. That's the power of body shape, and it's as easy as knowing the difference between apples and pears.

BODY SHAPE VARIATIONS

As much as we would like to believe that we are all unique physical specimens, women's bodies are divided into two main groups: apple-shaped and pear-shaped. The classic apple-shaped woman has slender and shapely legs, narrow hips, large breasts and a relatively large waist. If you look at an apple, you'll notice that the fruit is widest in the middle. An apple-shaped woman also tends to put on weight around her middle, that is, her waist, or the area where her waist would be if she had one. She probably owns few, if any, belts, but short skirts and men's-fit or slim-leg blue jeans look good on her. The classic pear-shaped woman has a relatively thin upper body, often with small breasts, a well-defined waist and a heavier lower body. If you look at a pear, you'll notice that the fruit is widest at the bottom. Again, a pear-shaped woman also tends to put on weight around her bottom – hips, thighs and buttocks. She may feel self-conscious about her 'thunder thighs', but she'll have no problem cinching a belt around her narrow waist.

Once you know what to look for, you can often identify which women are apple-shaped and which are pear-shaped just by looking at them. Spend a day people watching in a shopping mall and you'll see many examples of both classic apple shapes and classic pear shapes. You'll also spot a few mixed-type body shapes. For example, some women have more of a banana shape – a body that is straight up and down, with thin upper and lower extremities, small chest, and no waist. There is also a body shape sometimes called the 'inverted pear', characterised by large breasts and thick, wide shoulders tapering down to slender hips, but with no discernible waist. And, of course, there is the famous hourglass figure, defined by large breasts, a narrow waist and relatively large hips. Banana-shaped and inverted pear-shaped women have, for all medical purposes, variations of an apple shape. Women with an hourglass figure have the equivalent of a pear shape. All women, thin or fat, curvy or flat, can be categorised as either apple-shaped or pear-shaped. The key is the waist-to-hip ratio.

THE TAPE MEASURE TEST

Figuring out your body shape is easy – all you need is a flexible tape measure and a calculator. First, measure around your waist. If you have a visible waist, measure around the narrowest part. If you don't have a waist, measure around the widest part of your middle, usually about 3cm (1in) above your navel. Stand up straight, but relaxed. Don't suck in your gut. Hold the tape measure loosely, without putting pressure on the skin. That number is your *waist circumference*.

Next, measure around your hips – not where the bones of your pelvis jut out, but about 8–10cm (3–4in) lower. This actually corresponds to the point where the top of your thigh bone – the femur – meets the pelvis. You should be measuring around your buttocks, not above or below. If you have any doubt, take the measurement at the widest point of your lower body, which may include your 'saddlebags' if you are pear-shaped. Divide your waist measurement by your hip measurement to get your *waist-to-hip ratio*, or *WHR*.

If your WHR is 0.80 or lower, your body is classified as pear-shaped. If your WHR is higher than 0.80, your body is classified as apple-shaped. For example, if your waist measurement is 66cm (26in) and your hip measurement is 94cm (37in), then the calculation is 66 ÷ 94 = 0.70, which means that you are pear-shaped. If your waist measurement is 89cm (35in) and your hip measurement is 97cm (38in), then the calculation is 89 ÷ 97 = 0.92, which means that you are apple-shaped. It's that simple. But embedded in that simplicity is a whole new dimension of women's health.

ALL FAT IS NOT CREATED EQUAL

The essential difference between apple and pear shapes is fat – where it is, what type it is and how it affects health. It's not just a surface difference, like blond hair versus brown hair. It is a deep, fundamental difference; a genetic code that runs through every cell in our bodies coupled with hormonal variations.

Fat comes in two main varieties: *subcutaneous,* which means 'under the skin', and *visceral*, which means 'pertaining to the soft organs in the abdomen'. Subcutaneous fat is the stuff that jiggles, the soft stuff we pinch and poke and generally hate to see on our bodies. Visceral fat, on the other hand, is not always visible from the outside. It packs itself around the inner organs of the abdomen, jamming up against the intestines, kidneys, pancreas and liver (and sometimes even inside the liver). We all have some visceral fat because it protects our internal organs, acting both as shock absorber in case of trauma and as insulator to help us conserve body heat. While some visceral fat is necessary, too much can create serious health problems.

Fat comes in two main varieties: *subcutaneous,* 'under the skin', and *visceral,* 'pertaining to the soft organs in the abdomen'.

Most people think of fat as inert material, much like the rind of fat surrounding a good steak. If we cut it off (or suck it out, in the case of liposuction), all we're doing is getting rid of that hunk of congealed lard – right? Wrong. Fat is actually living, breathing, hormone-producing, metabolically active tissue. It is critical for survival, and not just because it provides storage for energy. Fat helps regulate body functions through the give-and-take of chemical communications with the central nervous system. People who have too little body fat are just as unhealthy as people with too much body fat, but in a different way. In fact, try not to think of body fat as *fat*. It's too easy to visualise a 'bucket of lard'. Instead, try to think of fat as a gland, as active and important as any other gland in the body. In medicine, we call fat 'adipose tissue', which has the benefit of reminding us that we're talking about an integrated part of the body, not simply dead weight.

Adipose tissues make and release a variety of compounds, including enzymes, hormones (such as leptin, which helps regulate appetite), and inflammation-related chemicals called cytokines. These and other factors, many of which have not yet been identified, come together to create your body's internal physiologic state. And what that state means for your health comes down to the type of fat you have. Although visceral fat and subcutaneous fat are in the same general category, they are totally different animals. To lump them together would be like saying that your eyes and your ears are the same because they are both sense organs. True, but the difference is as great as the difference between . . . well, sight and sound.

Fat helps regulate body functions through the give-and-take of chemical communications with the central nervous system.

Subcutaneous fat may be visible and annoying, but it is relatively harmless. Some of it may, in fact, help protect us from disease. Subcutaneous fat that collects around the *pear zone* – hips, thighs and buttocks – has been shown to increase levels of high-density lipoprotein (HDL, also known as the 'good' cholesterol) and actually helps maintain a steady balance of triglycerides in the blood. Subcutaneous fat in the pear zone is able to trap certain fats from the foods we eat, keeping them from escaping into the bloodstream, where they can damage our arteries.

Excess visceral fat, on the other hand, can be dangerous. Visceral fat is more metabolically active than subcutaneous fat, and most of what it does is harmful to the body. Visceral fat decreases insulin sensitivity (making diabetes more likely), increases triglycerides, decreases levels of HDL cholesterol, creates more inflammation and raises blood pressure – all of which increase the risk of heart disease. While fat in the pear zone traps and stores dietary fat (trapped fatty acids are then stored as triglycerides), visceral fat releases more of its free fatty acids into the bloodstream, further increasing the risk of both diabetes and heart disease. The overall effect of excess visceral fat is that it creates a physical environment that is primed for heart disease and stroke and greatly increases the risk for certain cancers. The more abdominal fat, the greater the waist circumference, and the higher the WHR, the more dangerous the situation becomes.

THE NATURE OF APPLES AND PEARS

The qualities of subcutaneous fat and visceral fat are different. And these fat differences are what make apple-shaped and pear-shaped women so varied in terms of how they look, their risk of disease and their metabolic activity. In many ways, these two categories of women are as physiologically different from each other as women are from men.

To nature, pear-shaped women are perfect – ideally designed for fertility, pregnancy, childbirth and long lives of nurturing. (Nature has a rather limited definition of 'perfect'.) Their body chemistry is dominated by oestrogen, that most female of hormones, which provides lush layers of back-up fuel – we call it fat – and protection around their eggs and womb. The pear shape is soft, curvy and warm, endowing women with distinct waists, hips, buttocks and thighs. In medical circles, the pear shape is known as 'gynoid', which derives from the Greek word for *woman,* as if all women were meant to be pear-shaped.

The apple shape is medically called 'android', which derives from the Greek word for *man.* In women, this means that their body chemistry is dominated by androgen, the typically male hormone. All women produce androgens in their ovaries and adrenal glands, but apple-shaped women produce more of them. They also produce oestrogen, of course, but there is a relative predominance of androgen helping to define how they look and function. The effect is that women with an apple shape have bodies that are shaped more like men's bodies – less curvy, more angular and with less fat around the lower body. They often have relatively large breasts, usually because of weight gain above the waist, coupled with the powerful way androgens affect the body.

If thin thighs, large breasts and a small bottom were the only outcomes of an android shape, there wouldn't be a problem. But there are repercussions. Apple-shaped women, with their extra androgens, tend to gain weight in the same way men do – around the waist, with much of it in the form of visceral fat.

So pear-shaped women and apple-shaped women not only look different, they *are* different. Apple-shaped women have the type of fat that promotes heart disease, whereas pear-shaped women have the type of fat that protects against heart disease. Apple-shaped women have decreased glucose tolerance, whereas pear-shaped women have steady glucose tolerance. Apple- and pear-shaped women react differently on a number of physiologic (and, as we'll see later, psychological) parameters, leading to varied disease risks. In some cases, apple- and pear-shaped women may respond differently to the same medications. Overall, the disparity between body shapes is so dramatic, it's as though we are looking at two entirely different groups of people.

Who Has the Greater Risk?

	Apple-Shaped Women	Pear-Shaped Women
Heart disease	√	
Type 2 diabetes	√	
Osteoporosis		√
Breast cancer	√	
Endometrial cancer	√	
Varicose veins		√
Stress	√	
Low self-esteem		√
Problems with body image		√
Eating disorders		√
Irregular menstrual cycles	√	
Menopausal symptoms		√

BODY TYPE IN HEALTH RESEARCH

The significance of this difference is staggering. When scientists do medical research, they usually lump all women together as a single category. Very few researchers separate women into two groups based on body shape. So when we read about a medical study of, say, heart attack in women, who are the researchers studying? Apple-shaped women? Pear-shaped women? A combination of the two?

The reality is that, in most cases, even the researchers don't realise the tremendous response differences between body shapes, so all women are studied as if they are identical. But as we've learned, apple- and pear-shaped women are not identical. They can even have exactly opposite physiologic responses to the same stimulus. So imagine what happens when a scientist studies a large group of women. The combined results of both body types could cancel each other out! Alternatively, the study may investigate the reactions of only one body type, purely by accident. In that case, results will be announced as pertaining to all women, when really only one type of woman was studied.

The result is that many health 'truths' that we take for granted *are not necessarily true for all women*. For example, we've heard that, statistically, men suffer more heart attacks than women. But a closer examination of the data reveals that apple-shaped women have the *same* heart attack risk as men when the amount of abdominal fat is taken into account. Pear-shaped women have a much lower risk of heart attack, regardless of their overall weight. In fact, virtually the only time a woman will have a heart attack before menopause is if she is apple-shaped or has diabetes . . . and 85 per cent of women with diabetes are apple-shaped! Study after study has shown that women who are shaped like men – apple-shaped women – are more likely to die like men, of the same causes and at the same rates.

Many health truths we take for granted are *not necessarily true for all women.* Women who are shaped like men – apple-shaped women – are more likely to die like men, of the same causes and at the same rates.

We know this because some astute physicians asked the question, Why do my female heart attack patients all seem to have an android fat distribution pattern? (We still didn't have the vocabulary to talk about apple-shaped body type back when these studies were being conducted.) The research provided what was then considered a surprising answer – that apple-shaped women had more heart attacks than pear-shaped women *simply because of their body shape,* and more specifically, because of the visceral fat that created that shape. Since then, most researchers have understood the importance of measuring waist circumference and (sometimes) waist-to-hip ratio in studies of women and heart attacks.

Although heart researchers may understand the importance of body shape, what about all the other women's health researchers? How confident can we be, then, with the universality of women's health research? When a particular study reveals, for example, that hormone therapy (HT, also called hormone replacement therapy) increases risk of heart attack in women (even when most doctors will tell you that their experience and years of observational studies tell them the opposite), how do we know which women were studied? Do the results pertain to all women, or just one category of women? Right now, we just don't know because the vast majority of research does not separate women by body shape.

The few intrepid researchers who have taken these differences between apple- and pear-shaped women into account are expanding the breadth of knowledge about women's health. The hope is that someday all women's health research will include the variable of body shape (through measurement of WHR and waist circumference) so that we have even more definitive prescriptive and preventive information. For now, we use what we have. And even though the research has really just begun, we already know enough about the differences between women with apple or pear shapes to make specific and customised health recommendations based on body shape, personal medical history and family history.

NOT ALL FRUIT SHAPES LOOK ALIKE

Although the extremes of body shape are easy to identify, there are many different varieties of apple shapes and pear shapes in the world. Total weight, in fact, has very little to do with it. Body shape is strictly defined by the waist-to-hip ratio. Notice the variety of apple and pear shapes in these photographs. Beneath each woman's picture are her shape category, WHR, and BMI (Body Mass Index).

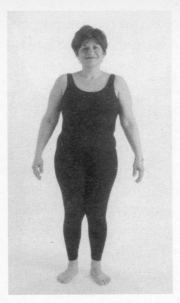

Apple
WHR: 0.85
BMI: 28

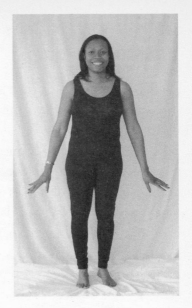

Apple
WHR: 0.88
BMI: 23

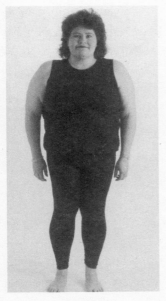

Apple
WHR: 1.05
BMI: 37

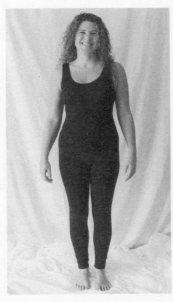

Apple
WHR: 0.82
BMI: 23

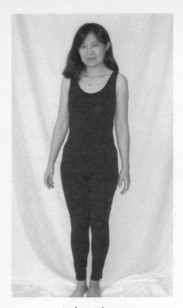

Apple
WHR: 0.82
BMI: 19.5

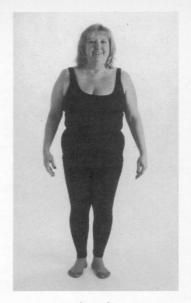

Apple
WHR: 0.89
BMI: 34

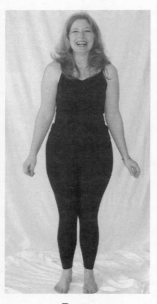

Pear
WHR: 0.72
BMI: 23

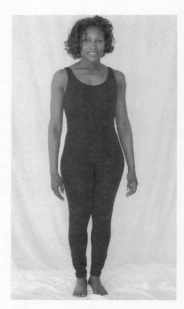

Pear
WHR: 0.73
BMI: 20

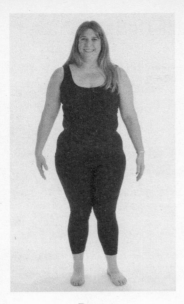

Pear
WHR: 0.78
BMI: 30

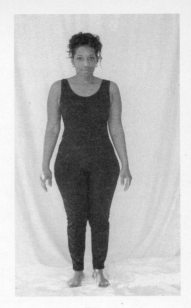

Pear
WHR: 0.72
BMI: 25

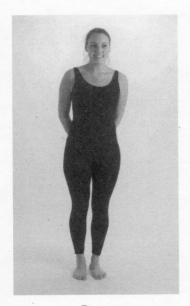

Pear
WHR: 0.73
BMI: 22.5

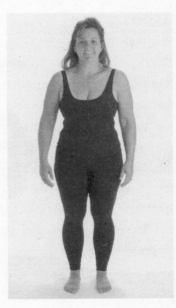

Pear
WHR: 0.76
BMI: 27

WHICH IS BETTER, APPLE OR PEAR?

Women seem to have preconceived notions of which body type is 'better', apple-shaped or pear-shaped. Each woman tends to think that whichever type she *isn't* is the more desirable. Pear-shaped women often silently curse their hips and thighs, dread swimming-costume season and can be embarrassed by their very womanly, Rubenesque figures. They have to fight the impression that they are wide at the bottom simply because they sit around all day – 'secretary spread' is a pejorative for ample buttocks on a woman with a desk job. Apple-shaped women are often uncomfortable with their bellies. They become geniuses at dressing to camouflage their lack of a waist and are often frustrated to tears at the inability of sit-ups or crunches to slim their middles. They feel shamed into making excuses for their shapes, such as blaming a large tummy on the effects of pregnancy 'baby weight' that never went away. (As you'll see in chapter 3, that's actually partly true.)

In reality, neither body shape is better than the other. It may sound as though science is picking on apple-shaped women, but apple-shaped women can be just as healthy as pear-shaped women. Everything depends on the amount of visceral fat they have. Shape, through waist circumference and WHR, is just a convenient way to measure that adipose tissue. So apple-shaped women can really consider themselves lucky to have such a good advance warning system for disease! Pear-shaped women may have less immediate disease risk, but they can become apple-shaped after menopause. And in old age, they face the quiet devastation of osteoporosis. There is no 'better' or 'worse', there is only what you are.

Regardless of whether you are an apple or a pear, fat or thin, it is important that you understand that your body shape is not your fault. And it is certainly nothing to be ashamed of. It's all part of the specific set of genes and environmental factors that make you who you are. Although scientists have begun mapping the human genome, it is likely that we'll never know exactly which other traits were inextricably interconnected and expressed to make you a unique individual. Are you creative, musical, funny, responsible, intuitive? Are you a great cook, a loving mother, a reliable friend? Are you happy, serious, playful, philosophical, strong? There's a good chance that the factors that went into making you those things are somehow linked to the factors that made you apple- or pear-shaped. You can't change it.

There is no 'better' or 'worse', there is only what you are. And your body shape is *not* your fault.

What you can do, however, is make yourself as healthy as possible. This includes identifying your body shape, recognising the inter-relatedness of body shape and certain diseases, and then doing what you can to rid yourself of excess visceral adipose tissue. Visceral fat is the enemy, not your waist, hips, thighs or bottom. This book is full of ways to get rid of visceral fat, prevent the additional accumulation of fat and counter some of the other disease risks associated with your body shape. Just take one step at a time. If you adopt even a few of the programme recommendations, you won't need a crystal ball to tell your health future – you'll see it in the mirror, and you'll feel it in your heart.

Action Items for Chapter 1: Apples and Pears

◆ Measure your waist circumference (WC) and your hip circumference, then calculate your waist-to-hip ratio (WHR) to determine whether you are currently apple-shaped or pear-shaped.

◆ Find the Body Shape Health Log for your shape, beginning on page 328, and write in your current measurements. It is going to be important for your health records to keep track of both your WC and your WHR. As you move forward with the diet and exercise programme customised for your body shape in Part 3 of this book, you'll want to monitor your progress by updating these numbers periodically. The logs have spaces to track other health numbers, which I'll explain as we go along.

Take to Heart . . .

◆ Being apple-shaped is not inherently good or bad. Being pear-shaped is not inherently good or bad. Is it better to be a beagle or a cocker spaniel? A rose or an orchid? If you understand and accept your body type, you will gain the freedom to be happy in your own skin.

CHAPTER 2
Weight and Body Shape

It would be impossible to miss the message that obesity is now epidemic throughout the world. During two weeks in February 2004 alone, American and British newspaper headlines proclaimed: DOCTORS CALL FOR ACTION OVER OBESITY 'TIMEBOMB'; KILLER HABITS 'NEED URGENT ATTENTION'; FAT 'THE NEW TOBACCO', HEART GROUP WARNS; ALARM SOUNDED ABOUT RISING RATE OF OBESITY IN KIDS. The phenomenon is so far-reaching that the World Health Organization has coined a new word for this devastating health crisis: 'globesity'. We know that obesity is related to an increase in an individual's risk of heart disease, stroke, type 2 diabetes and the metabolic syndrome, and many types of cancer, not to mention gall bladder disease, osteoarthritis, depression and gum disease. It slows us down, adds to back pain, makes it difficult to breathe, and generally reduces our quality of life. But how do we determine who is obese and who is not?

Although it seems like a simple question, medical professionals have debated the best ways to define 'obese' for decades. Human beings are not as easily categorised as you might suspect. We have variations of height, bone mass, muscle tissue and other factors that make our degree of fatness difficult to gauge. Nevertheless, a person is generally considered to be obese if she is carrying 25 per cent more weight than is considered optimal for good health.

Sure, individuals, cultures, societies and professions all have different standards and definitions of overweight. But in the world of medicine, definitions become important if we want to help people identify their specific risks and take action to avoid the diseases related to fatness. The debate is still going on. Should we measure straight body weight, or is a calculation of weight by height more accurate? Some health professionals use calipers to pinch and measure the skin folds in certain areas of the body. Others will weigh a person on dry land, then dunk her in a pool of water and weigh her again. Because body fat weighs less in water than on land, a simple calculation can reveal what percentage of the body is fat and what percentage is lean muscle mass.

Now, the burgeoning issue of body shape has added a new wrinkle to that old debate, and it raises an interesting question: Do all kinds of obesity contribute to health risks, or just visceral obesity?

WEIGHT AND BODY MASS INDEX (BMI)

Most of us are familiar with the concept of body weight. We stand on the scales and learn how much our body weighs in kilograms or stone and pounds. I'll wager a guess that you know your current weight (within a kilo or two). Most women do. It's a rare woman who can't tell me not only what she weighs today, but what she weighed in secondary school, in college or university, before and after having children and on her last birthday. We've been trained over the last three decades to incorporate weight into our sense of self and, too often, self-worth. I can't tell you how many times I've told friends that they look terrific, and they replied with some version of 'Well, I'd look better if I could only lose five pounds'. As if they didn't deserve a compliment because of their extra weight. Incredibly, some of my women patients have told me that they delayed making an appointment for a physical exam because they wanted to lose weight first . . . or worse, they didn't schedule the physical at all because they couldn't lose the weight they knew they needed to lose, which I learned only if we happened to be standing in the same supermarket queue! We pin so much of our sense of 'goodness' and 'success' on our current weight that we overlook the ultimate goal: good health.

Body mass index (BMI) was developed to acknowledge that a person's weight is related to her height. Rather than measuring weight on its own, the BMI is a score that standardises kilos/pounds-per-height. The scores are grouped into ranges that reflect who is 'underweight', 'ideal', 'overweight' or 'obese'. BMI allows us to see our place in the weight spectrum at a glance.

To find your BMI, find the row for the number closest to your weight on the vertical axis on the left side of the chart on page 22. Draw a light pencil line across that row, through all the numbers. Next, find the column for the number closest to your height on the horizontal axis at the top of the chart. Draw a light pencil line down that column, through all the numbers. The number in the box where the two pencil lines meet is your BMI. If your number falls in the shaded area (BMI 18.5 to 24.9), your weight is considered 'ideal'. If your number falls above the shaded area (BMI below 18.5), you are considered underweight; if your number falls below the shaded area (BMI 25 and higher), you are considered overweight. If your BMI is 30 or higher, your degree of overweight is called 'obese'. (Please remember that that word – obese – is not a judgment, it is a scientific label.)

Although BMI is more stable and a better indicator of fatness than weight, its main weakness is that it doesn't take muscle mass into account. A lean, muscular bodybuilder has a dense, heavy body, and therefore can have a BMI that defines her as overweight even though her body fat is minimal. Still, BMI is the primary measurement used by researchers to define 'overweight' and 'obese' for clinical studies. Although health experts recommend that doctors use BMI to diagnose patients and recommend treatment, they rarely use it. Most women don't know or remember their current BMI number. That's probably because

BMI CHART

Weight (kg) \ Height (cm)	150	152	155	157	160	163	165	168	170	173	175	178	180	183	185	188	190
40	18	17	17	16	16	15	15	14	14	13	13	13	12	12	12	11	11
45	20	19	19	18	18	17	17	16	16	15	15	14	14	13	13	13	12
50	22	22	21	20	20	19	18	18	17	17	16	16	15	15	15	14	14
55	24	24	23	22	21	21	20	19	19	18	18	17	17	16	16	16	15
60	27	26	25	24	23	23	22	21	21	20	20	19	19	18	18	17	17
65	29	28	27	26	25	24	24	23	22	22	21	21	20	19	19	18	18
70	31	30	29	28	27	26	26	25	24	23	23	22	22	21	20	20	19
75	33	32	31	30	29	28	28	27	26	25	24	24	23	22	22	21	21
80	36	35	33	32	31	30	29	28	28	27	26	25	25	24	23	23	22
85	38	37	35	34	33	32	31	30	29	28	28	27	26	25	25	24	24
90	40	39	37	37	35	34	33	32	31	30	29	28	28	27	26	25	25
95	40+	40+	40	39	37	36	35	34	33	32	31	30	29	28	28	27	26
100	40+	40+	40+	40+	39	38	37	35	35	33	33	32	31	30	29	28	28
105	40+	40+	40+	40+	40+	40	39	37	36	35	34	33	32	31	31	30	29
110	40+	40+	40+	40+	40+	40+	40	39	38	37	36	35	34	33	32	31	30
115	40+	40+	40+	40+	40+	40+	40+	40+	40	38	38	36	35	34	34	33	32
120	40+	40+	40+	40+	40+	40+	40+	40+	40+	40	39	38	37	36	35	34	33
125	40+	40+	40+	40+	40+	40+	40+	40+	40+	40+	40+	39	39	37	37	35	35
130	40+	40+	40+	40+	40+	40+	40+	40+	40+	40+	40+	40+	40	39	38	37	36
135	40+	40+	40+	40+	40+	40+	40+	40+	40+	40+	40+	40+	40+	40	39	38	37
140	40+	40+	40+	40+	40+	40+	40+	40+	40+	40+	40+	40+	40+	40+	40+	40	39
145	40+	40+	40+	40+	40+	40+	40+	40+	40+	40+	40+	40+	40+	40+	40+	40+	40
150	40+	40+	40+	40+	40+	40+	40+	40+	40+	40+	40+	40+	40+	40+	40+	40+	40+

BMI is abstract – it doesn't stick as easily in the mind, and it's difficult to visualise what one might have to do to go from an unhealthy BMI of 31 to a healthy BMI of 24. For these reasons, researchers tend to use BMI in their studies of obesity and its effects, while women and their doctors (for the most part) continue to measure and talk about pure weight.

HOW BODY SHAPE FITS IN

Medical researchers have recently discovered that weight and BMI are only part of the health equation. Studies have shown that measurements of waist circumference and waist-to-hip ratio (WHR) are more predictive of future disease risk than your weight or BMI. For example, the respected Iowa Women's Health Study showed that obese women with a high WHR (apple-shaped women) had a 20 to 50 per cent higher risk of death from all causes (depending on which other risk factors were included in the calculation) than obese women with a low WHR (pear-shaped women). In other words, the critical factor was body shape, not obesity.

Measurements of waist circumference
and waist-to-hip ratio are more predictive of future
disease risk than weight.

The closer you read the medical research literature, the clearer this message becomes. For example, diabetes researchers have discovered that signs of prediabetes – low glucose tolerance and high insulin levels – are found more often in individuals who have large amounts of abdominal fat, but not in those who are generally obese or who have large amounts of subcutaneous fat. In another study of nearly 12,000 Dutch women, those with the highest WHR (apple-shaped) were more than three times as likely to develop type 2 diabetes, more than twice as likely to develop high blood pressure, and had double the risk of developing gall bladder disease compared with women with the lowest WHR (pear-shaped), regardless of total weight. A Swedish study found that women with large hips (pear-shaped women) had less risk of heart disease and diabetes than women with small hips, again *regardless of total weight.*

One fascinating study of the power of body shape on metabolic risk involved identical twins. As you probably know, identical twins share all the same genetic material, which makes them ideal research subjects because any differences between them will be due to personal differences, not to any hidden genetic factor. This study looked at 23 sets of twins in which one twin was fat and the other was lean. The researchers separated the set of twins into two groups. One group was for twins where the fat twin had primarily subcutaneous fat (pears), and the second group was for twins where the fat twin had primarily visceral fat (apples). The researchers then checked to see whether the type of fat affected insulin sensitivity, insulin levels and glucose levels – measures of metabolic abnormalities. They found that abnormalities occurred only in those who had large amounts of visceral fat, *not* in participants who had large amounts of subcutaneous fat. Then, the researchers compared each fat twin to his or her lean twin to determine whether the metabolic abnormalities were due to genetics or to fat. If the fat and lean twins both had the same metabolic abnormalities, then the difference would be due to genetics. If one twin had a metabolic abnormality but the other did not, then the difference would be due to fat. The findings? Twins with visceral fat had significant metabolic abnormalities – higher levels of glucose and insulin and lower insulin sensitivity – compared with their lean twin. However, the twins with high subcutaneous fat had metabolic results that were virtually identical to those of the thin twins. This means that overweight pear-shaped twins were just as metabolically healthy as the lean twins! So it wasn't *all* fat that caused metabolic abnormalities and therefore increased their risks of diabetes and heart disease, it was only the visceral fat. This tells us that people who are apple-shaped and overweight are more likely to have metabolic abnormalities caused by their excess fat than any other group. However, it's important to note that lean apple-shaped twins had normal metabolism – good health was within reach just by losing weight!

WAIST CIRCUMFERENCE TO REFINE THE RISK

One of the most definitive and comprehensive studies of the effects of body shape on disease risk is the Nurses' Heath Study, which followed more than 120,000 female nurses for more than 25 years, looking at all possible risk factors for heart disease. As part of this study, researchers looked at the relationships among BMI, waist circumference, WHR and risk of heart attack. They found that both waist circumference and WHR were better predictors of heart attack than BMI, with WHR being the best measure of the three. Specifically, this study showed that middle-aged apple-shaped women are more than twice as likely to have a heart attack as pear-shaped women, *regardless of body weight*. This unfortunately means that even apple-shaped women with relatively low body weight have a relatively high risk of disease. Pear-shaped women generally have lower risk of heart attack across the board, even if they are overweight. In fact, in this study the pear-shaped women with the highest BMI still had lower rates of heart attack than apple-shaped women with the lowest BMI.

A Danish study published in 2003 echoed these findings. It showed that among postmenopausal women, those who were overweight with a pear shape had less risk of heart disease than overweight *and lean* apple-shaped women. Lean apple-shaped women still have a much lower risk of heart disease than overweight apple-shaped women, but pear-shaped women just happen to have an added advantage in that their pear-zone fat seems to protect them from many of the diseases associated with visceral fat. This might seem frustrating to apple-shaped women, but please try to remember that you are not in a health 'race' with other women, you're only competing against yourself. Your personal risk of type 2 diabetes and heart disease gets worse if you gain weight and gets better if you lose weight, so at least that part of your health is in your control.

In a second analysis, the Nurses' Health Study demonstrated that overall waist circumference is a strong and independent disease predictor. The researchers discovered that the larger the waist, the greater the risk of heart attack, such that every centimetre you add to your waist incrementally increases your risk of heart disease. This makes perfect sense. A larger waist means that there is more of the dangerous visceral adipose tissue, so the danger of heart attack is greater, too. Other studies have had similar results, showing that waist circumference measurements are better than BMI when it comes to predicting weight-related diseases, including hypertension, the metabolic syndrome and type 2 diabetes.

The larger the waist, the greater the risk of heart attack. Every centimetre you add to your waist incrementally increases your risk of heart disease.

This means that risks for all diseases increase with greater 'appleness'. If you have an apple shape with a WHR of 0.85, then you have less of a risk than a woman with a WHR of 0.95, or 1.15. Although pear-shaped women are relatively protected, their risk also increases with every additional centimetre on their waists. This, too, makes sense. Although pear-shaped women tend to put weight on around their lower bodies, some abdominal fat will also be gained. So while they may have less of a risk than apple-shaped women, pear-shaped women also face increased risks as their waist size grows.

HEALTH BY THE CENTIMETRE

The accumulation of data tells us that for many of the most debilitating and dangerous diseases it is not all fat that contributes to disease risk, just visceral fat. Therefore, *it is not weight we need to worry about, but centimetres.*

Weight isn't everything.

Let me repeat that, because I think a lot of women are going to have trouble grasping such an odd and alien concept: stop worrying about your weight. Concentrate instead on your waist measurement. In fact, I don't want you to worry about weighing yourself at all. Your doctor will take care of that at your next medical visit. If you own scales, hide them in the back of your messiest cupboard, toss them in the attic or give them away. Don't succumb to the temptation to define yourself by your weight anymore. If you reduce the size of your waist, you can't help but lose weight, but to me, the change of focus is critically important. How many years have you gone on diet after diet trying to lose weight? Let's break the cycle of failure and start fresh. Let's work on your waist. And while we're doing that, let's also work on other health changes you can make and specific actions you can take to lower your risks of disease even before you budge the first centimetre off your waist. Weight isn't everything. The programmes in this book transcend kilos, stone and pounds and I'll walk you through what you need to know and what you need to do, step by step.

It is not all fat that contributes to disease risk, just visceral fat. So, stop worrying about your weight. Concentrate instead on your waist measurement.

For apple-shaped women, then, the question becomes one of degree – how much visceral or abdominal fat is normal and how much is dangerous excess? The current guidelines (for those of you who like guidelines) are that women with a waist circumference greater than 88cm (34½in) should actively work to lose abdominal fat. This is generally considered the 'cut-off' for good health. However, lower waist circumferences have been shown to be even more protective, and women are encouraged to try to get their waist circumference down to 81cm (32in) or less. One study even suggested that a woman can't consider herself at a 'safe' size until she reduces her waist to below (30in).

One major drawback to these guidelines is that they were developed based on research using middle-class Caucasian women. Subsequent research has shown that different ethnic groups have different body shapes and different health risks that require different waist circumference guidelines. It's important to remember, however, that for all ethnic and racial groups, the higher the waist circumference, the higher the disease risk. Only the precise cut-off numbers are being investigated. Unfortunately, this research is only in its beginning stages. What we know so far is:

◆ Chinese and Asian Indian women develop metabolic problems and heart disease at lower waist circumferences than do Caucasian women, so the guideline for their optimal waist size is smaller. How much smaller is not yet known, but a cut-off of 81cm (32in) has been suggested, with a possible optimal measurement of 71cm (28in).

◆ Hispanic and Mexican women experience greater risk of diabetes and hypertension at lower waist circumferences than Caucasian women and therefore need a lower cut-off. More research needs to be done before appropriate guidelines can be offered.

◆ African-American women have about twice the rate of obesity compared with Caucasian women. They also have lower insulin sensitivity (a bad thing) and greater risks of heart disease and diabetes. Interestingly, studies have shown that African-American women tend to have less visceral fat and more subcutaneous fat compared with Caucasian women at the same total body weight. This is confusing to everyone, and more research needs to be done to figure out all the factors that might be contributing to the obesity-related health risks of African-American women. One interpretation that has been suggested is that African-American women might have a greater sensitivity to the effects of visceral fat compared with Caucasian women, so that even lesser amounts of visceral fat equate to worse risk outcomes for African-American women. Still, it is clear that visceral fat is harmful to the health of African-American women, and they should be encouraged to reduce waist size.

THE FIVE-CENTIMETRE RULE

Personally, I'm not a fan of specific waist circumference guidelines. If you are close to having a 75cm (30in) waist, then maybe the guidelines will work to motivate you to try just a little harder to meet that goal. If that works for you, use it! But many women in the developed countries of the world haven't seen a 75cm (30in) waist since they were in their teens (if then). I don't want this to become another case of setting impossible standards. For those of you who have a waist circumference considerably larger than 90cm (35½in), please remember that these guidelines are formed by researchers who are setting ideal standards in an artificial environment. If you were my patient, I would tell you to *concentrate on losing just 5cm (2in) off your waist.* You are allowed to forget the guidelines and work on your own personal, customised plan.

Reducing the waist measurement has been shown to reduce total cholesterol, reduce low-density lipoprotein (LDL – the 'bad' cholesterol) and reduce blood pressure. In fact, research shows that women who lost just 5cm (2in) off their waists were able to improve at least one major risk factor by 10 per cent or more. Although 10 per cent may not sound like much, it is a significant and important change when it comes to cardiovascular benefits. A mere 5 to 10 per cent change in body weight can mean a lower LDL cholesterol and higher HDL cholesterol, an improved insulin sensitivity, a reduction in inflammation markers (see chapter 6 for more information about inflammation markers) and a decreased risk of blood clots and stroke. A measly 10 per cent change in any individual risk factor is enough to bring many people out of the 'danger zone' for diabetes and heart disease. *Every centimetre* of abdominal fat you lose will significantly decrease your risk of diabetes and heart disease and very possibly add years to your life. And that is my greatest wish for you.

The good news is that your body *wants* to get rid of excess visceral fat. It is the first kind of fat you'll shed, so you'll be getting healthier right away from the first day you start your programme.

If you are one of the millions of women who now know that they need to work on reducing their waists, the body shape programmes in this book will help you do exactly that. If you are overweight, you will also lose kilos – but that is not my overall goal for you. If you are already at your ideal weight but want to narrow your waist, you will shed fat and lose girth, but you may or may not lose weight. Fat loss doesn't always equal weight loss. The good news is that your body *wants* to get rid of excess visceral fat. It is the first kind of fat you'll shed, so you'll be getting healthier right away, from the first day you start your programme.

BODY SHAPE IN THE DOCTOR'S SURGERY

Has your doctor ever measured your waist during a physical exam? Most likely not. And yet patients are often weighed as part of a health check. We know that waist circumference and body shape are much more powerful predictors of future health than straight body weight – so why aren't they used?

Some doctors claim that it takes too much time to have a patient undress and measure a waist, or that it is too embarrassing if the patient is a woman. (Here's an idea – make waist measurement part of your next appointment for a cervical smear or a mammogram. The tape measure won't seem nearly as embarrassing compared with the stirrups!) Doctors, too, fall victim to embarrassment or time constraint issues. An editorial published in the February 24, 2003, issue of the *Archives of Internal Medicine* stated: 'Many physicians are more comfortable ordering a plasma insulin level and prescribing insulin-sensitizing medications than measuring a waist circumference and discussing diet and physical activity.'

Another reason why waist circumference and WHR have not made their way into medical offices is that there's no money to be made by preventing disease with an inexpensive tape measure. Pharmaceutical and medical device companies would rather develop and promote expensive laboratory tests than support measuring health 'by the inches'. This is one area of medicine that disappoints me – we seem to do everything possible to avoid giving power to the person who needs it the most, the patient. I have been outspoken on this issue for quite some time. To me, measuring and monitoring your waist circumference is a classic example of a way to regain control over your health because it is predictive, simple and empowering.

When the need for medical cost control reaches a critical level, chances are that more basic, less expensive tests will prevail. I predict that it is just a matter of time before the tape measure test becomes a standard part of every physical examination, as critical a vital sign as blood pressure is today. Until then, it's up to you to use the knowledge at your fingertips to make yourself as healthy as possible. The next time you visit your doctor, tell her your waist circumference and WHR. Talk about your plan for reducing your waist size to improve your health so that you will have a health professional on your side. Your doctor should be thrilled to help in any way possible.

Action Items for Chapter 2: Weight and Body Shape

◆ Throw away or hide your scales. The goal is to stop measuring your health by weight and begin measuring your health by changes in your waist circumference, and possibly your WHR. It's not that I don't care about obesity, but I'd like to encourage you to start thinking about your risk of disease from the perspective of body shape, not weight.

◆ If you don't already own a flexible tape measure, go out and buy one. They are available in haberdashery departments, and they usually cost less than a cup of gourmet coffee.

◆ Once you have a tape measure, hang it on a hook in your wardrobe or bathroom so that you can measure your waist once a month during the programme. In the meantime, having the tape measure hanging where you are likely to see it when you are nude or dressing is a nice visual reminder that you are now practising health by the centimetre, not by the kilo.

◆ Measure your waist. *If you are an apple-shaped woman,* subtract 5 from that number and write the result on an index card or other small piece of paper. Pin up that number someplace where you can see it daily – on your mirror, in the top drawer of your night table, on the refrigerator. The mind has a tremendous effect on the body. By pinning up your goal number, you are priming your mind to make the changes that will help you lose centimetres. *If you are a pear-shaped woman,* look at the BMI chart on page 22. If your BMI is 25 or higher and your waist circumference is greater than 90cm (35½in), then follow the instructions for apple-shaped women above. (This pertains only to this action item. Apple- and pear-shaped women will have different recommended programmes for waist reduction.) If your BMI is less than 25, then you may not need to reduce your waist size. It will be more important for you to concentrate on the overall health maintenance portion of the programme for pear-shaped women.

Take to Heart ...

◆ Knowing your body shape is more helpful than knowing your weight when it comes to your future health. Take this opportunity to think for a moment about the freedom that will come from never having to step on the bathroom scales again, and the joy that will come from being able to accept yourself as a woman with a figure, instead of as a body with a weight problem.

CHAPTER 3

Shape-Shifting
with Life Transitions

O ur bodies are constantly changing. The dramatic physical metamorphoses women experience across their lifetimes prove that we are geniuses of accommodation and flexibility. Only chameleons change more than we do. The greatest leaps in our personal evolution occur at specific life stages, those physiologic windows of opportunity that forever alter the way our bodies function and look. The first occurs at puberty. All children start out apple-shaped, and boys stay apple-shaped. But once the hormones of adolescence hit, girls can either remain apple-shaped or become pear-shaped. For most women, pregnancy marks the next great change, followed by menopause and, if we're lucky, old age.

As you read about each of these life stages, you'll notice that nature seems determined to make apples of us all. Women who are already apple-shaped may see their waistlines expand, but not quite understand that each extra centimetre means more than just tight-fitting jeans. Pear-shaped women may find that their body shape changes entirely. They can end up confused and frustrated, living in an apple-shaped body that feels foreign.

All children start out apple-shaped, and boys stay
apple-shaped. But once the hormones of adolescence
hit, girls can either remain apple-shaped or become
pear-shaped.

None of us was given an owner's manual at birth, so we don't usually know what to expect or how to respond to the changes that come upon our bodies. Many of us simply allow life to happen. We become like rudderless boats on the sea, helpless in the face of winds and tides. It doesn't have to be that way. By understanding how life stages affect body shape, you can gain the freedom to make the kinds of positive choices that will steer you away from health disasters.

CHILDHOOD AND ADOLESCENCE

Our health as adults depends in large part on our weight and fitness levels as children. The body sizes and shapes of tomorrow's adults are being formed in today's children.

One of the jobs of a growing body, along with developing muscles and lengthening bones, is to form fat cells. These fat cells have many different functions, but one of their primary roles is to keep us from starving. If we run out of immediate fuel in the form of food, fat stores break down to supply the body with the energy it needs to keep going. If we eat more calories than we burn off, then the excess energy (because a calorie is a unit of energy) is stored as fat. It doesn't just get dumped like so much toxic sludge – fat gets neatly stored in our fat cells. Think of them as tiny balloons that store all those extra calories until we need them.

With a couple of important exceptions, by about age 21 we generally have a full complement of fat cells, at which time the body stops actively making them. That means that when we gain weight as adults, we don't typically create new fat cells, we just fill the fat cell balloons we already have. Where the fat cells are located depends on the body shape we've developed – apple-shaped women have more fat cells located deep in their abdomens, and pear-shaped women have more fat cells at their hips, thighs and buttocks.

As the fat cells fill with fat, they start expanding, just like a balloon. When the cells reach their capacity, the body gets the message that the storage units are full, and new fat cells are created. (This is one of the exceptions to the 'no more fat cells' rule.) This certainly fixes the storage problem, but it is not an optimal solution. You see, when we lose weight, fat cells get smaller, but they never go away – unless they are removed by liposuction. Scientists have discovered that the more fat cells you have, the more difficult it is to lose weight. And even if you are successful, having more fat cells makes it more difficult to keep the weight off. Why? Remember, the job of a fat cell is to store fat. It hates being deprived. Imagine that you have lost 10kg (1 stone, 8lb). You are happy because your clothes fit better, but your fat cells are feeling empty. When the amount of fat in your fat cells drops significantly, those cells will try to stop the fat-loss process by sending out signals that they need to replenish their stores of fat. Those signals will act on your brain by making you want to eat – fat cells produce hormones that help regulate appetite – or on your body by making it conserve energy. The main way the body conserves energy is to lower metabolism.

All those fat cells don't want to be depleted, so they conspire to conserve all the fat they have. That's why 85 per cent of people who lose weight put it all back on again within about a year.

If you think of your metabolism as a campfire, lowering metabolism is like dousing that fire and lighting a match instead. A healthy metabolism 'fire' burns off calories from food and from stored fat if it runs out of available calories. A lower metabolism burns fewer calories, which means more fat gets stored in fat cells. The result is that you end up gaining back those 10kg (22lb) you lost. You don't even have to start overeating to regain the weight – the regular amount of food your 'normal' metabolism could handle is too much for your lower metabolism. That's why about 85 per cent of people who lose weight put it all back on again (and then some) within about a year. All those fat cells don't want to be depleted and conspire to conserve all the fat they have.

So all the way from babyhood through adolescence, we are naturally increasing the number of fat cells in our bodies. If a child becomes overweight, the number of fat cells increases even more, and they may end up with more fat cells than an adult of average weight. These kids are put on the road to a lifetime of hard-to-fight obesity right from the start. And we're talking about a lot of little lives . . . it is heartbreaking. In November 2004 it was estimated that 10 per cent of all six-year-olds and about 17 per cent of all fifteen-year-olds in Britain were obese (with a BMI over 30).

The consequences are frightening. Type 2 diabetes used to be called 'adult onset diabetes' because it was virtually unheard of in younger populations. Now, diabetes is being diagnosed in children as young as age seven. These children risk developing obesity-related diseases earlier in their lives, which means that they will spend their adulthoods battling not only diabetes, but cardiovascular disease, cancer and a host of other health difficulties. The psychological toll is also a concern. As difficult as it is to be an overweight adult in our society, life is even harder for overweight children. In a study published in 2003 in the *Journal of the American Medical Association,* researchers found that, compared with healthy children, obese children and adolescents had impaired functioning in all domains of life – physical, emotional, educational and social – due to their obesity. How badly does obesity affect the well-being of a child? This same study found that the quality of life of obese children was rated *the same as the quality of life of children with cancer,* a group that had been thought to have the worst emotional consequences.

If you were an overweight child then I don't have to explain any of this to you. I'm sure you remember the social stigma and emotional pain quite well. I only mention this in a book about apple and pear shapes because a young overweight girl is more likely to develop into an apple-shaped woman, with all its physical ramifications. As a 2003 British study showed, not only are children becoming heavier and heavier, but their waist circumferences are increasing at an even faster rate than their BMI. So it appears that overweight children are not just putting on fat, they are putting on mostly visceral fat. Researchers have raised the concern that putting on too much visceral fat in childhood might actually impair the development of fat in the pear-zone. Being overweight might override a girl's genetic programming and make her apple-shaped instead of pear-shaped. We may be raising a generation of apple-shaped women who won't have the benefit of the health protection given by lower-body fat.

PREGNANCY AND BODY SHAPE

There are two main questions we can ask when looking at this life transition: (1) how does pregnancy affect body shape; and (2) how does body shape affect pregnancy?

How Does Pregnancy Affect Body Shape?

Pregnancy – that most female of physical states – paradoxically seems to help create an android or apple-shaped body. Studies have shown that women who have never been pregnant have lower waist-to-hip ratios (making them more pear-shaped) than women who have had one or more children. And when researchers looked at individual women, taking their measurements before and after pregnancy, they found that weight gained or retained after pregnancy seems to be mainly visceral fat. Although no one really knows why this happens, there are several factors that all seem to help push pregnant women towards appleness.

Pregnancy is one of those times when your body naturally starts adding fat cells – making it the second of the exceptions to the fat cell rule. In an average pregnancy with a weight gain of 14kg (2 stone, 2lb), about 3 of those kilos (7lb) go directly to increasing the mother's fat stores. That is considered a healthy and necessary amount of weight to support the stress of the physical post-partum period. Much of it can be lost through diet, exercise and breastfeeding (which burns a lot of calories), but research shows that the average woman permanently retains between 0.5 and 3.6kg (1–8lb). In addition, many women find that pregnancy becomes a trigger for additional weight gain – so although they may have maintained a normal weight all their lives until pregnancy, those women keep gaining for months or years after the baby is born. Some women can continue gaining in excess of 18kg (2 stone, 12lb). And a large percentage of that weight is in the form of dangerous visceral fat.

For many women, bearing children changes the
contours of their bodies forever.

No one knows exactly what makes some women more likely to gain or retain weight after pregnancy. There is a disagreement in the literature about whether prepregnancy weight has any effect, with some researchers saying that obese women gain or retain more weight after pregnancy, and other researchers saying that prepregnancy weight makes no difference. Other studies report racial differences: Caucasian women are more likely to gain pregnancy-related weight if they are young and already overweight; but African-American women are more likely to gain pregnancy-related weight if they are older and of normal weight. Why? Again, we don't know. These are some of the questions that have yet to be answered by medical science.

The overall point is that for many women, bearing children changes the contours of their bodies forever. A pear-shaped woman won't turn into an apple-shaped woman, but her waist might never again be quite as small as it was before pregnancy. My own experience after two pregnancies and three children (a set of twins!) was that my total body weight didn't change very much, but my waist became larger and I could no longer fit into jeans that I had worn comfortably before the pregnancies.

How Does Body Shape Affect Pregnancy?

As of this writing, there haven't been any published studies that look at the effects of body shape on the amount of weight gain after pregnancy, but it wouldn't surprise me if apple-shaped women retained more weight than pear-shaped women. That's because researchers have discovered that apple-shaped women have high insulin levels during pregnancy more often than pear-shaped women. High insulin levels are known to cause weight gain, so this may cause apple-shaped women to add several kilos above the average weight gain of pregnancy. Apple-shaped women also have a greater risk of developing gestational diabetes, which is not surprising. Developing gestational diabetes is a risk factor for the later development of type 2 diabetes, and we know that apple-shaped women are more likely to develop type 2 diabetes than pear-shaped women. All this is saying is that apple-shaped women run a higher risk of metabolic problems throughout their lives, including during their younger childbearing years.

In addition, apple-shaped women have a higher risk of developing high blood pressure and pre-eclampsia (high blood pressure along with protein in the urine and/or significant fluid retention) during pregnancy. Although the greatest risk is for women who are both apple-shaped and overweight, at least one study showed that even lean apple-shaped women have an increased risk of pre-eclampsia compared with pear-shaped women.

Please remember that although an apple shape increases your risk of gestational diabetes and pre-eclampsia, it doesn't mean that you are destined to have problems during pregnancy. Simply knowing about these connections gives you an added edge so that you can monitor your blood pressure and blood glucose more carefully and get help early if you develop either condition. Dietary changes are also important. I believe that any apple-shaped woman – especially if she has a family history of diabetes, pre-eclampsia, the metabolic syndrome or large babies – should work with a dietitian before becoming pregnant, or as soon as the pregnancy is recognised. And I'd like to reassure all women, pear-shaped and apple-shaped, that there is no reason to avoid the joys of pregnancy and child-rearing just because of the risk of additional visceral fat. Yes, body changes come with the motherhood territory, but the programmes in Part 3 can help you minimise any negative effects of the added girth. The important thing is to be aware that it can happen, and that it may change the way you have to think about and monitor your health.

Remember the story of my mother in the Introduction? She kept putting more and more weight around the middle after each child – she had eight of us in all – but she didn't realise the dangerous effect this slow and steady weight increase was having on her heart. She didn't change her health habits until after her heart attack. If you stay aware of any post-pregnancy-related changes to your waist circumference, and follow the programmes later in this book, you will be able to prevent or delay the diseases related to visceral fat.

MENOPAUSE AND AGEING

As we get older, our tendency to put on weight around the waist increases. This is just as true for men as it is for women. Year by year, body weight slowly increases, with an average weight gain of between 0.5 and 1kg (1–2lb) per year. We also tend to lose lean muscle mass and replace it with fat, in part because we become more sedentary and less active. This is important because muscle tissue is much more metabolically active, weighs more and burns more calories than fat. So if a woman gradually loses muscle mass throughout her life, her metabolism will slow down and she will be more inclined to put on weight as she gets older. The only way to preserve lean muscle mass is to remain active; we will not lose muscle if we continue to work out. When my babies were little, I had a very strong upper body from carrying all three up and down stairs, one piggyback and one in each arm. I got stronger and stronger as they grew from infants to young children . . . my muscles grew as they grew! When I stopped carrying them, I lost my arm muscles. A true case of 'Use it or lose it'.

The only way to preserve lean muscle mass is to remain active. We will not lose muscle if we continue to work out.

As we get well into our 40s and older, menopause seems to want to make apples of us all, mainly because of our plunging oestrogen levels. At puberty, the oestrogen rise puts fat preferentially around girls' hips, bottoms, and thighs, turning many of them from baby apples to young adult pears. The opposite happens after menopause. As women undergo the transition from premenopause to post-menopause, waist circumference increases and hip circumference decreases, speeding the conversion from pear-shaped to apple-shaped.

This shift happens even if there is no additional weight gain. The body just reshapes itself. After menopause, lean muscle mass decreases more dramatically, and a larger proportion of weight gain becomes visceral fat. Total body fat and visceral fat both continue to increase throughout the ageing process, so that the longer a woman lives after menopause, the more apple-shaped she will become.

REMAINING STRONG AND HEALTHY FOR LIFE

When it comes to body shape, the natural course of change is all in one direction – towards the apple. Each major life transition leaves souvenirs for us to remember it by: the breasts and hips of adolescence, the stretch marks and fuller waist of pregnancy, the gradual fattening after menopause. These changes are not controllable, even by the most dedicated of us. Just as you couldn't stop your breasts from developing when you were an adolescent, you also can't fight many of the physical changes after pregnancy and menopause. I like to think of these shape-shifting alterations as having my body renovated by an eccentric but creative architect. I may not know exactly what the final outcome will look like, but I'm certain that it will be unique.

That doesn't mean that we are entirely powerless. There are decisions we are allowed to make, and our choices will be reflected in our health 10 to 50 years from now. We can't prevent all the changes, but we can offset their effects by adopting a habit of healthier eating, regular physical activity, not smoking, moderate alcohol use and attending to medical needs.

We need to pay *more* attention to our health as we
get older, not less.

I've noticed that there is a tendency for some women to decide at some point along the life trail that it's just not worth the effort to try to fight the fat any more. They have the idea that healthy eating and exercise are for those who are young and already thin, probably because there are few good fitness role models for women who feel overweight or over-the-hill. Oprah Winfrey is a remarkable exception. Her continuing and very public efforts to make her body healthy and strong – marked by successes and setbacks – have been inspirational to millions of women who relate to her struggles. The bottom line is that we need to pay *more* attention to our health as we get older, not less. Caring for yourself shouldn't stop just because you are busy, or because you turned 50, or you got married, or you had a baby. In Part 3 of this book, I outline the paths that will help you become the healthiest you can be, *at any point in your life*. I give you the tools you'll need to fix or improve many of the unhealthy changes that might have come upon you during a life-stage transition. You may still make poor choices now and again, but at least you'll have enough information to make an informed decision. Every woman – young or old, apple-shaped or pear-shaped, fat or lean – has unlimited chances to become stronger and healthier. It is never too late.

Action Items for Chapter 3:
Shape-Shifting with Life Transitions

◆ Knowing your body shape – and the forces that helped create it – gives you a perfect opportunity to size up your current health status. On one side of a piece of paper, write down all your major life transitions and critical turning points in the order in which they happened. Begin with the start of menstruation, and include all physical and emotional milestones you've had, including gradua-tions, marriages, divorces, pregnancies, serious diseases or medical conditions, menopause, death of a loved one, or anything else that is significant to you. All these life events and transitions, physical and emotional, have had an effect on your body. Take a moment to reflect on how those events affected you physically. Did you gain weight? Lose weight? How did your body shape change? Did you become ill or depressed? Look at how much your life has changed and how your body responded to those changes throughout the years. You have so much experience with change – you can't possibly doubt that you can make positive changes now!

◆ On the other side of that same piece of paper, write down all the major diseases or disorders that you are currently being treated for. Then, draw a line, and below it write down all the major diseases or disorders that run in your family. Finally, at the bottom of the page, write down the disease that scares you the most. This is your inventory of health concerns. Most people feel helpless in the face of disease, but you don't have to just take what comes. In Part 2, I discuss how body shape is related to many of the most frightening and serious diseases. Then, I explain the best steps towards preventing, reversing, delaying or treating those conditions. Knowledge gives you the power and the confidence to face down your health fears.

Take to Heart ...

◆ We are all destined to pass through life's stages; we can't turn back the clock. But for every loss, each life stage brings us joys, as well – the love of our children, the freedom and independence that comes with menopause. Do your best to live in the moment so you can enjoy each stage as it comes along.

◆ If you are feeling guilty about 'losing your shape' after childbirth or menopause, let it go. Some of the changes in your body are inevitable and uncontrollable. But that doesn't mean that you have to put up with the unhealthy consequences of those changes. We'll work on improvements together.

PART TWO
MEDICAL ISSUES

CHAPTER 4

The Hormone Question: From Childbearing Years to Postmenopause

Hormones produced in the human body are some of the most powerful substances on Earth. The smallest amounts – applied at the right time and in the proper combinations – can act as a love potion, weight-loss drug, fertility enhancer, appetite suppressant, appetite stimulant or immunity booster. They can give us energy or make us sleepy, make us grow breasts or beards, speed up our metabolism or slow it down to a crawl. Body shape is most influenced by the hormone insulin and the sex hormones: the 'female' hormones *oestrogen* and *progesterone,* and the 'male' hormones collectively known as *androgens.*

The sex hormones kick in at puberty, fluctuate in regular monthly cycles during our menstrual years, and then trickle to a halt at menopause. Body shape is related to the relative dominance of sex hormones. A woman with a 'gynoid' or pear shape has a predominance of female hormones, whereas a woman with an 'android' or apple shape is more greatly influenced by male hormones. I don't want any

49

misunderstandings – apple-shaped women are fully, 100 per cent female. The amount of male hormones in an apple-shaped woman is nowhere near the amount found in the average man. But even a little extra androgen can have far-reaching effects. We already know that apple-shaped women have a body fat distribution that is more typically masculine, and that their risk of heart disease is the same as men's risk (at the same levels of visceral fat). These same hormones, the 'apple' hormones, have other effects that run throughout women's lives.

HORMONE BASICS

As you might expect, having more of the male-dominant hormone means that apple-shaped women can face challenges with reproductive body functions. Compared with pear-shaped women, apple-shaped women tend to have more menstrual irregularity and more problems with infertility. Apple-shaped women also have an increased risk of blood clots or heart problems when taking birth control pills, and they have a very difficult time tolerating hormone therapy (HT). For this reason, apple-shaped and pear-shaped women may need to take different paths when it comes to birth control or menopause treatment.

To appreciate these differences, it's important to understand the overall hormone mix. Let's start with a look at a typical, and highly simplified, sequence of hormones during the menstrual cycle.

1. As eggs in the ovaries begin to grow (developing eggs and their surrounding 'nests' are called *follicles*), they start to produce small amounts of oestrogen.

2. As one or more eggs mature before ovulation, higher amounts of oestrogen are released by the ovary.

3. When oestrogen levels get high enough, they cause other hormones in the body to be produced, which in turn cause ovulation so that the follicle bursts and the fully mature egg is released. The ruptured follicle produces both oestrogen and progesterone. These hormones remain at high levels in the body until menstruation, when production drops and a new cycle begins.

Progesterone is the unsung hero of this little drama. It makes only a brief appearance each month, but it is critical for regulating the length of the menstrual cycle and maintaining the hormonal balance in the uterus. Progesterone is first produced by the follicle that releases the egg and remains the main hormone guiding the final two weeks of the menstrual cycle. It contributes to the maturation of the lining of the uterus in preparation for a fertilised egg and pregnancy. Some women with extremely short menstrual cycles are thought to have inadequate progesterone production, and treatment with progesterone can sometimes correct menstrual cycle irregularities, excessively heavy bleeding or between-period spotting.

A woman's reproductive health depends on balance among all the hormonal forces in her life. When prescribing HT after menopause, doctors know that giving oestrogen alone can cause a build-up of the uterine lining, which can lead to endometrial cancer (cancer of the uterine lining). HT needs to include both oestrogen and progesterone to maintain the balance.

Pear-shaped women generally have their hormones in balance, which creates an ideal environment for pregnancy. They have regular periods, are more fertile and tend to ovulate like clockwork. Even the fat they carry around their lower body is a special preparation for childbirth. For pears, it's 'all systems go', all the time. Until menopause, of course. Then the hormonal picture changes.

In contrast, the extra androgens in apple-shaped women throw off their hormonal balance. For example, small amounts of additional androgens can suppress ovulation. Not all the time, but sometimes. That's one of the reasons apple-shaped women have more problems with fertility. Women who don't ovulate regularly don't always go through all three stages of the simplified hormone cycle listed above – they go through stage 1 and stage 2, but without ovulation, they don't get to stage 3. And stage 3 is where progesterone is produced. That means that oestrogen remains unbalanced. (Physicians use the term 'unopposed', which conveys the notion that oestrogen is in there having effects without any counteracting or balancing force.) If this happens often enough, apple-shaped women end up with *too much oestrogen* and *not enough progesterone*. Without the balance of progesterone, apple-shaped women face an increased risk of endometrial cancer.

Nature has provided a clear model of the effects of too much androgen in women: polycystic ovary syndrome (PCOS), a genetic disorder that causes excess production of androgens. It is estimated that 5 per cent of women have PCOS, with a higher prevalence among Italians, Hispanics and Ashkenazi Jews. Women with PCOS don't ovulate. With an ultrasound, we can see that their ovaries are full of cysts that are unruptured follicles – ripe eggs that were never released from the ovaries. Women with PCOS often experience irregular or infrequent periods, with particularly heavy bleeding when they do arrive. The higher-than-usual levels of male hormones can cause excess body hair, acne, a deeper voice or even male-pattern baldness. These symptoms can be severe, but they are usually mild enough that women with PCOS often don't have a clue that anything is wrong until they seek medical treatment for infertility.

Most significantly, women with PCOS tend to put on visceral fat, have a high risk of type 2 diabetes, an increased risk of heart disease and an increased risk of endometrial cancer. Sound familiar? This is similar to the health pattern we see in apple-shaped women. In fact, many apple-shaped women have PCOS without knowing it. But please don't panic if you have an apple shape and acne or an abundance of leg hair. PCOS is a clinical diagnosis that must take into account medical history, physical examination, ultrasound of the ovaries (to look for cysts) and blood tests to measure hormone levels. It is not something you can tell just by visual examination, and no single test can confirm or rule out PCOS. Plus, the overall health effects are not much different from those of an overweight apple-shaped woman. Treatment usually involves taking hormones (in the form of birth control pills) to regulate menstruation, and perhaps other medications if diabetes, high cholesterol or hypertension is also present. If you have PCOS, the recommendations for apple-shaped women in this book are exactly right for you, too.

HORMONES BEFORE MENOPAUSE

When young women make the decision to take oral contraceptives instead of other forms of birth control, they are usually thinking about the low failure rate and general convenience of the Pill. Indeed, the Pill is the most effective birth control method available, and it has been used by millions of women safely for decades. In addition, it confers some noncontraceptive benefits. There is usually an improvement in acne, which can be significant for some women. The Pill prevents iron-deficiency anaemia because the combination of oestrogen and *progestin* (the synthetic form of progesterone) leads to a much thinner uterine lining and therefore a lighter period or less bleeding. And contraceptive hormones can also suppress benign ovarian cysts and minimise or lessen fibrocystic breast symptoms. Most important, taking the Pill reduces a woman's risk of ovarian and endometrial cancer. Still, it is a more complicated decision than many women think.

Most oral contraceptive pills in use today are a combination of oestrogen and progestin. Although we think of oestrogen as the power-house hormone, the truth is that the progestin is really the active ingredient in birth control pills because it does three things that prevent pregnancy: (1) prevents ovulation; (2) makes the natural cervical mucus thicker so it becomes an impenetrable barrier for sperm; and (3) thins the lining of the uterus so even if ovulation happens to occur, and even if sperm actually get to it, the egg can't become implanted and therefore cannot develop. The oestrogen is really only added to balance out the excess progestin. Again, balance is key.

The typical pill cycle is three weeks of hormone pills, followed by one week of placebo pills. (The new brand Seasonale gives you 12 weeks of hormone pills, with one week of placebo pills.) The hormone pills put the body in a kind of steady state where nothing is really happening, fertility-wise – there is no ovulation and no menstruation. During the week of hormone-free placebo pills, the abrupt cessation of hormones leads to the sloughing of the lining of the uterus – what we know as menstrual bleeding.

As you might expect, given their differences in hormone levels, fertility and menstrual regularity, apple- and pear-shaped women have different needs when it comes to hormone-related birth control, or 'premenopausal hormones'. But the possible side effects and complications apply to both body types. Any woman over age 35 who smokes should not take the Pill because of the increased risk for heart attack, stroke and blood clots. Other women who should not take the Pill:

◆ Women who have a family history of breast cancer, because it is thought that oral contraceptives might contribute to breast cancer in women who have the BRCA1 or BRCA2 genes;

◆ Women who suffer from migraine headaches, because the headaches often get worse on the Pill, and there may be an increased risk of stroke in some migraineurs;

◆ Women who carry one of the high-risk human papillomavirus (HPV) strains, because the Pill may increase the chances of cervical cancer in these women – ask your doctor to test for these strains if you are age 30 or older, or if you have an abnormal smear test result.

Others at risk for life-threatening side effects are women with risk factors for cardiovascular disease – especially women with diabetes, high blood pressure, high cholesterol, high C-reactive protein (CRP, a marker of inflammation tied to heart attack risk), a history of blood clots or phlebitis (inflammation of veins in the leg) – *and overweight apple-shaped women.* Some studies have shown that women who take oral contraceptives may have an increased risk of developing insulin resistance, which could potentially trigger type 2 diabetes. Apple-shaped women have a higher risk of insulin resistance and diabetes by virtue of their body shape and visceral fat stores. So apple-shaped women need to be very careful about the types of birth control hormones they choose in order to avoid triggering health problems. All the more reason to understand the risks and benefits, to consult with your physician or health care practitioner, and to choose the best options for *you*.

Birth Control Recommendations for Apple-Shaped Women

For apple-shaped women who need birth control, or women with PCOS who need to stabilise their menstrual cycles, I recommend:

1. **The 'patch'.** The Janssen-Cilag Evra transdermal birth control patch (norelgestromin with ethinyl oestradiol) is my first choice for apple-shaped women. It is a combination of the lowest possible oestrogen dose, with a form of progestin that has low androgenic (male hormone) activity. The patch and all combination oral contraceptive pills contain the potent oestradiol form of oestrogen – only the progestin varies. Norelgestromin is a progestin with low androgenic activity, which is better for apple-shaped women who are already dealing with excess androgens. Even better, the patch is applied to the skin, so that the hormones are absorbed at a slower, more even rate. The skin route also means less risk of complications because the drugs bypass the liver, which means that you'll need

less hormone in your body to get the same effect. Compared with oral contraceptives, the patch will also cause less of a rise in dangerous triglycerides, the storage form of fat in our fat cells. The transdermal patch seems to lower total and low-density lipoprotein cholesterol (LDL, the 'bad' one), with no change in high-density lipoprotein cholesterol (HDL), triglycerides, or C-reactive protein (CRP), which means that there is less of an increase in heart disease risk compared with oral contraceptives. It also lowers the risk for high blood pressure, migraine headaches and their complications, and blood clots. But although the transdermal route may be safer, I still do not recommend any form of hormones to women with a history of phlebitis, blood clots or pulmonary embolism. Another downside is that the patch is not fully effective if a woman weighs more than 90kg (14 stone, 2lb) because the dose of hormones is just not enough to guarantee ovulation suppression.

2. Low-androgenic pill. Yasmin (drospirenone with ethinyl oestradiol), or Cilest (which include the norgestimate-containing progestins with ethinyl oestradiol) contain a form of progestin that has the lowest androgenic activity. Yasmin is my choice for women with PCOS because it directly blocks the testosterone side effects, such as excess body hair and acne. These pills, like all oral oestrogens, increase levels of C-reactive protein (CRP) and raise risk of heart disease and blood clots.

3. Progestin-only pills. I recommend Micronor (norethindrone), and Microval (levonorgestra) progesterone-only pills for women who need a reliable birth control method but cannot take oestrogen, such as women with many cardiovascular risk factors or prior blood clots. These hormone options avoid oestrogen, and therefore may not increase the risk of blood clots, cardiovascular disease and stroke. They also stop excessive bleeding, which can be a problem for some apple-shaped women. They do not, however, treat excess hairiness or acne (you need the addition of oestrogen to do that), so they are not a good choice for women with PCOS who take the pill primarily to treat their androgen symptoms. On the other hand, progestin-only pills are perfect for women with PCOS who have no menstruation and need to bring on a cyclic period every few months to prevent unopposed oestrogen and a build-up of uterine lining.

Birth Control Recommendations for Pear-Shaped Women

Although oral contraceptives are generally safer for pear-shaped women than for apple-shaped women, there are still some guidelines. First, pear-shaped women who smoke forfeit their natural health advantages, so they should not use hormone-based contraception after age 35. Second, pear-shaped women aged 35 and older who have high risk of heart disease or blood clots also shouldn't take the pill.

For pear-shaped women younger than 35, contraceptive hormones are incredibly safe. They can take their pick of using the Janssen-Cilag Evra transdermal patch or taking any of the available pill formulations. My first recommendation is usually the patch for women who like the convenience of not taking pills (see description above on page 55). For women who prefer pills, I recommend a low-dose combination pill, such as Cilest (with 35 micrograms of oestrogen, for young women who need higher doses to suppress ovaries) or Loestrin 20 (with only 20 micrograms of oestrogen, for older women who need less hormone to suppress ovulation – less is always better). Although some pills are advertised as being better for women with acne, almost any combination oral contraceptive pill will lessen acne by reducing androgen levels.

Pear-shaped women tend to have very regular menstrual cycles, but too much weight loss can upset the balance of hormones. As a result, very small, thin women, such as ballet dancers or women with eating disorders, often stop ovulating or ovulate erratically. Thin pear-shaped women who don't have regular cycles should have their hormone levels evaluated. If they have low oestrogen and progesterone levels, then they *need to start taking oral contraceptive pills* – not only for birth control, but to provide oestrogen for their bones and general health, and progesterone to keep the hormones balanced. Pear-shaped women who are overweight may have irregular menstrual cycles due to other physical problems, such as thyroid disease. They should always have a thorough physical examination to determine the source of the problem.

HORMONES DURING PERIMENOPAUSE

About 5 to 10 years before a woman goes into full-fledged menopause, her ovaries begin to fail and she may start to experience symptoms from the decline of oestrogen. This intermediate time is called peri-menopause. Her periods may become shorter, longer or irregular. She may experience weight gain (heralding even greater potential weight problems after menopause), irritability, mood swings, hot flushes, sleep disruption or changes in libido. It can feel like premenstrual syndrome . . . but it can also feel like symptoms of menopause.

Too many times doctors try to offer relief by prescribing hormones to women in the perimenopause. Doctors often prescribe oral contraceptives, even if a woman has had a tubal ligation and is not at risk for pregnancy. The pills may relieve the perimenopausal symptoms, but because the women are older, they have an increased risk of the typical hormone contraceptive complications. Alternatively, doctors may prescribe low doses of the same HT given to women in menopause. These hormones are not strong enough to suppress ovulation, and you can imagine the surprise felt by many women who were taking the lower-dose HT in their late 40s or early 50s and then discovered that they were pregnant.

The decision to take medication is an individual one, based on your body shape, your personal and family health history and the symptoms you would like to treat. I still do not routinely recommend oral contraceptive pills to women older than age 35, and I don't think that perimenopause symptoms are a good reason to make an exception. Oral contraceptives are much stronger than menopausal HT.

Perimenopause Hormones for Apple-Shaped Women

Apple-shaped women are less likely to have problems with the low-oestrogen symptoms caused by perimenopause, so I don't recommend oestrogen – especially not potent oral contraceptive pills. However, apple-shaped women in the perimenopause are more likely to have heavy bleeding and erratic periods. Even though they ovulate less, they continue to build the uterine lining from oestrogen, but now they have much less progesterone to balance it out, so they bleed. Perimenopausal apple-shaped women with symptoms of progesterone drop (heavy bleeding and erratic periods) without symptoms of oestrogen drop (such as hot flushes, mood swings or night sweats) can take progestin-only medication, such as Prometrium, a natural progesterone. You take it for 10 days every 3 months to bring on a bleeding cycle and 'clean out' your uterus to prevent endometrial cancer.

Perimenopause Hormones for Pear-Shaped Women

Pear-shaped women have a greater tendency to experience symptoms of low oestrogen during the perimenopause compared with apple-shaped women. Using the same HT as menopausal women really isn't an option. It isn't strong enough to suppress ovulation, so not only will pregnancy be a risk, but bleeding may also be erratic and unpredictable. Most oral contraceptives, however, are too strong. If low-oestrogen symptoms are intolerable, I recommend that pear-shaped women try taking Loestrin 20, the oral contraceptive with the lowest possible dose of oestrogen. Still there may be some hidden health risks. Many perimenopausal pear-shaped women I know – myself included – have tried the lowest dose of oral contraceptive, but our blood pressure rose dangerously high. If you can't tolerate Loestrin 20, try the alternatives discussed at the end of this chapter. If they don't work, a final possibility is to try a natural progesterone, either in prescription pill (Prometrium) or gel (Crinone) form, or in over-the-counter cream. I have seen lots of women find some relief of perimenopausal symptoms by using the cream, but there is no support for its use in the scientific literature. Most research shows that the creams have no more benefit than a placebo. Still, we know that progesterone can be absorbed through the skin, so it may very well work for some subset of women that hasn't yet been defined. The problem is that it's difficult to know how much progesterone is really being absorbed, so the results will vary from woman to woman. If you want to try natural progesterone cream, I recommend asking your pharmacist to mix up a batch just for you. This will ensure that a certain verifiable amount of progesterone will actually be in the cream. If you prefer to buy a packaged cream, look online for the brand Pro-Gest, which has the longest and best track record, and use as directed on the package.

HORMONES FOR MENOPAUSE AND BEYOND

After menopause the ovaries shut down and stop producing oestrogen and progesterone. But that is not the end of the hormone story. Oestrogen can still be present in our bodies in three different ways:

◆ Oestrogen is typically stored in body fat, so a woman who is overweight at the time of menopause will still be carrying stores of oestrogen that can serve her well for many years.

◆ Body fat – that metabolically active adipose tissue – has enzymes that can change androgens into oestrogen. It's important for women to realise that visceral fat and gynoid fat create different forms of oestrogen. Visceral fat converts androgen into oestradiol; gynoid or pear-zone fat converts androgen into oestrone, a much weaker form of oestrogen. Oestradiol and oestrone both have the same general properties, but oestrone is less potent. So apple-shaped women will have more oestrogen after menopause than pear-shaped women because their visceral fat will convert their extra androgens into the potent oestrogen.

◆ We can take hormone therapy, adding oestrogen from the outside.

Body shape is key to understanding how your health will be affected by menopause.

> Visceral fat and gynoid fat create *different forms of oestrogen.* Visceral fat converts androgen into oestradiol; gynoid or pear-zone fat converts androgen into oestrone, a much weaker form of oestrogen. Oestradiol and oestrone both have the same general properties, but oestrone is less potent. So apple-shaped women will have more oestrogen after menopause than pear-shaped women because their visceral fat will convert their extra androgens into the potent oestrogen.

Pear-shaped women who are thin or of normal weight have the worst hormone-related problems after menopause because they will naturally have the lowest levels of oestrogen. They have virtually no oestrogen stores (because they have relatively little body fat) and minimal amounts of androgens to convert to oestrogen. The oestrogens that are produced will be the weaker oestrone form. Because oestrogen is one of the main factors that protect our bone mass, thin pear-shaped women have the highest risk of developing osteoporosis. Plus, pear-shaped women usually experience the worst transition through menopause – worse hot flushes, insomnia, irritability and other symptoms.

Pear-shaped women who are overweight have fewer health risks after menopause than their thin counterparts because they have a larger oestrogen storage area (the extra pear-zone fat) and because the extra weight helps maintain bone mass simply by the pressure applied to bones by the extra kilos. As a result of the oestrogen stored in fat, overweight pear-shaped women tend to have moderate symptoms at menopause.

After menopause, pear-shaped women of all sizes lose their oestrogen advantage, and can therefore start to experience many of the same health problems as apple-shaped women – especially increased risks of heart disease and diabetes. Before menopause, pear-shaped women gained weight in their hips, buttocks and thighs first because of the predominance of oestrogen. When they gain weight after menopause, the tendency is to put on visceral fat instead of gynoid fat because of declining oestrogen; if enough visceral fat is acquired, body shape can transform from pear into apple.

I can't begin to tell you how many of my menopausal friends tell me their body has changed. They point to their newly acquired 'spare tyre' around their abdomen or note that they can no longer wear belts. The good news is that when women of any shape lose weight, the fat around the middle is the first to go. That's because visceral fat is metabolically easier to access compared to subcutaneous fat. It's like the difference between keeping your clothes in the wardrobe in your bedroom, or locked in a trunk in the attic – when you need a blouse, which location are you more likely to go to? Visceral fat is the easier location for the body to go to when it needs fat to burn, so when you lose weight, your waist tends to shrink first. In fact, it is extremely difficult for pear-shaped women to lose weight from their hips and thighs. So a pear is a pear, until she becomes an apple – but she can always transform back again with the right combination of diet and exercise. HT will help preserve the pear shape by adding back the missing oestrogen, and therefore reducing the tendency to put on visceral fat after menopause.

The good news is that when women of any shape lose weight, the fat around the middle is the first to go.

In general, apple-shaped women have fewer hormone-related problems after menopause than do pear-shaped women. The same extra androgens that gave them their apple shapes are still around after menopause, and androgens are converted to oestrogen. And because apple-shaped women have more visceral fat, the oestrogen that is made is the more powerful oestradiol. Therefore apple-shaped women tend to have a much easier menopause transition than pear-shaped women, with fewer hot flushes and other symptoms. Plus, they have a much, much lower risk of osteoporosis. (Finally some good news for apples!)

But after menopause, apple-shaped women, regardless of their weight, need to continue to monitor their health. Diabetes and heart disease continue to be major risks. With just a little extra attention to diet, exercise and other lifestyle choices, apples can be just as healthy as pears.

THE CONTROVERSY OVER HORMONE TREATMENT

In the mid-1990s, an extensive study in the United States called the Postmenopausal Estrogen and Progestin Interventions (PEPI) Trial, funded by the National Institutes of Health, reported what was considered the final word on HT – hormones kept women from gaining weight after menopause, strengthened bones and protected their hearts by reducing the risk factors for cardiovascular disease. Then, in 2002, a large and impressive study called the Women's Health Initiative (WHI) showed that HT could actually be harming women by increasing their risks of breast cancer and heart disease. Subsequently, the Royal Colleges of Obstetricians and Gynaecologists published a book warning of the dangers of long-term use of HT. Once the news hit the media, many women stopped HT, even as their doctors cautioned them not to overreact. Women were left with confusion and fear about what taking HT might have done to their bodies. Those with extreme, debilitating symptoms from menopause were caught in a damned-if-they-did, damned-if-they-didn't dilemma. Take hormones to feel 'human' again but risk disease down the road, or stop taking hormones and suffer the unbearable physical consequences of menopause.

The final word on the safety and efficacy of hormone therapy for menopausal women is not in. The data are still not clear. In 2003, 25 of the world's top hormone therapy experts gathered to discuss and debate the merits of the WHI study and the future of HT. The outcome was simple and refreshing. The experts decided that the WHI study – the one that caused millions of women to stop taking HT – looked at the effects of HT on *women who should never have been taking HT to begin with*. For example, more than 20 per cent of the women in the study were aged 70 or older, ages for which most physicians would not even consider hormone therapy. This makes the overall results suspect. Consider also that the body mass index (BMI) of most women in the WHI study was in the overweight to obese range, *and* that women with hot flushes (most likely the pear-shaped women) were discouraged from participating in the study. (This group was discouraged because HT definitely abolishes or lessens hot flushes, so these women would know by their symptoms whether they were taking HT or the placebo.) In addition, the average age of women who participated was 63 years, many had diabetes and hypertension, and some even smoked. These women had a good 10 to 15 years of menopause with little or no oestrogen. If you consider that most women who seek out HT do so because of unbearable hot flushes, and that apple-shaped women tend to have few, if any, hot flushes, *and* that women after menopause who don't take oestrogen become more apple-shaped, then the women in this study were most likely *overweight apple-shaped women*. This is one of those cases where the results of the study are not necessarily true for all women, only for older women who are overweight and apple-shaped.

Incidentally, those 25 international experts, after reviewing and discussing all the available data, recommended that hormone therapy 'should be given to women with menopausal complaints to meet their individual needs, taking into account their individual risk profile and the overall therapeutic objectives'. That's a fancy way of saying that it is an individual decision, between a woman and her doctor, based on family and personal medical history. I agree. I would never want any woman to make such an important medical decision based on a single scientific study or even a single book, including this one. Below, I give my HT recommendations for apple-shaped and pear-shaped women, and some alternatives you may not have considered. But this information is intended to educate you; it is not a prescription. Every woman is different, and important medical decisions should only be made by an informed individual in conjunction with her doctor. Just be warned that some doctors have a one-size-fits-all approach to HT, so learn all you can, go into the surgery armed with information, and get what you need. Ideally your doctor will be flexible and up-to-date, and will be happy to adapt your regimen to your unique circumstance.

HORMONES AND BREAST CANCER

We have known for years that taking oestrogen for five or more years increases a woman's risk of breast cancer. Recent studies have confirmed this increased risk. Most medical professionals believe that oestrogen doesn't *cause* cancer, but that it serves as fuel to a potential cancer that is microscopically small. If cancer is present, then adding oestrogen may make it grow faster. Unfortunately, the studies of breast cancer and hormones haven't looked at the effects of body shape. There may be differences in how pear-shaped and apple-shaped women respond to oestrogen in the breast. For example, it has been shown that apple-shaped women, who have higher oestrogen concentrations throughout their lives, have higher overall risk of breast cancer. Adding still more oestrogen after menopause might differentially increase their risk even further. We just don't know. And we have no idea about whether the risks are different for pear-shaped women.

We know the increased risk for breast cancer exists. The next questions are: How much does the risk increase, and what does it mean for you? In the WHI study of 2002, women who took combined oestrogen plus progestin had no increased risk of in situ breast cancer (early and noninvasive) and a 26 per cent increased risk of invasive breast cancer. And the risk seems to increase with the number of years a woman is taking HT. Currently, most guidelines suggest that HT not be taken for longer than five years because of the increased cancer risk. Women who have had a hysterectomy are eligible to take oestrogen alone, without the progestin. Oestrogen alone does not seem to significantly increase the risk of breast cancer.

What does this mean for you? If you have a family history of breast cancer – especially if you carry the BRCA1 or BRCA2 breast cancer genes – you should probably avoid taking hormones. If breast cancer frightens you more than any other disease, you should probably avoid taking hormones. Even though the overall increased risk is small, some women feel that any risk is not worth it. If that is you, stay away from hormones. Still, you should know that all experts agree that any woman could safely take HT for a year or two – the clinically significant increased risk for breast cancer doesn't begin until after five years of use.

HT Recommendations for Apple-Shaped Women

Several years ago, I treated a patient who was a physician's dream – informed, health conscious and determined to try to do everything right. Rhonda was also a mildly overweight classic apple, with the typical large chest, wide waist and thin legs. She came to see me because there had been many stories in the news about the cardiovascular benefits of being on HT. This was back in the 1990s, before the controversy. Because Rhonda had a family history of early heart disease, she wanted to start taking hormones to reduce her risk.

After more than 20 years in medical practice, I understood intuitively that women who hold their weight around their waist and higher (I didn't even think to categorise them as apple-shaped back then) didn't tolerate hormones well. They 'blow up' – their breasts become swollen and painful, their abdomens become distended and they bleed heavily during the monthly cycle that is reinstated by the hormones. Still, every woman is different. Rhonda wanted to be healthy. She had read all the latest medical reports about how hormones were good for heart risk, and she had a known family history of cardiac disease. So although I had concerns, I gave her a prescription for oral hormones.

Within days, Rhonda phoned my office. She felt absolutely miserable. Her breasts felt like overinflated balloons that could pop at any moment. Her abdomen felt bloated and she felt premenstrual, with all the attendant tension and agitation. But she wanted to persevere. She figured if she could wait out the first month, her side effects would get better. They didn't. She began vaginal bleeding within days, rather than at the end of the first cycle – and her bleeding was frighteningly heavy. She gave up on hormones almost immediately.

In retrospect, I see that I could have anticipated the way Rhonda's body would react, how uncomfortable she would be. Not only that, but with what I understand now, I realise that because of her apple shape she was exactly the wrong person to give hormones to.

Overweight apple-shaped women
should not take HT.

Right from the start, before I explain why and give you some alternatives, I want to tell you that overweight apple-shaped women *should not take HT*. It is likely that the hormones will *increase* your chances of having a heart attack, *increase* your risk of having blood clots or a stroke and *increase* your risk of breast cancer. They may also increase your risk of diabetes by reducing insulin sensitivity. And that's if you can get past the bleeding, bloating and other unpleasant side effects. Apple-shaped women have spent their lives living with an imbalance of oestrogen and excess androgens. After menopause, their excess androgens are converted into the more potent form of oestrogen. And their bodies are already saturated with oestrogen. Moreover, if an apple-shaped woman is overweight at the time of menopause, her extra body fat will contain even more oestrogen. When apple-shaped women take *more* oestrogen in the form of HT, their tissues get bigger in response to the extra hormone, and they end up bloated, like Rhonda.

This is a complex issue. Research has confirmed that taking hormones tends to protect postmenopausal women from accumulating stores of visceral fat. Remember, oestrogen puts on the pear-zone fat in the first place, beginning at puberty. With declining oestrogen at menopause, pear-zone fat gradually disappears. Without oestrogen, the body stores fat in the abdomen, so a pear-shaped woman can turn into an apple-shaped woman. By taking HT, which replenishes the oestrogen, a pear-shaped woman can preserve her pear shape. Apple-shaped women will never become pear-shaped, but over time, the dwindling supply of oestrogen will tend to cause them to become *more* apple-shaped. But for most apple-shaped women, HT does more harm than good.

Although taking hormones is theoretically beneficial, HT also:

◆ raises levels of triglycerides – and apple-shaped women may already have perilously high triglycerides, a danger sign for diabetes and heart disease;

◆ lowers insulin sensitivity by at least 30 per cent – and apple-shaped women already have a risk of lowered insulin sensitivity, the first step toward diabetes; and

◆ raises blood levels of C-reactive protein (CRP), the marker of inflammation that often warns of heart disease – and apple-shaped women already have higher levels of CRP, and higher risk of heart disease.

Plus, remember that most apple-shaped women have fewer symptoms at menopause . . . so why should they *want* to take HT? Based on this scientific research, and on my personal experience treating women, I no longer recommend HT to most apple-shaped women – especially if they are overweight or have a waist circumference larger than 90cm (35½in). (If you are an apple-shaped woman and you are currently taking hormones, don't stop taking them without informing your health care provider. You'll want to taper down according to medical instructions. Moreover, because many women feel uncomfortable side effects when they discontinue the medications, you'll want the support of your doctor.)

Thin apple-shaped women can take HT, but I really don't recommend it unless their symptoms are intolerable. Again, the decision of whether to take HT is highly individual. HT will bring back vaginal lubrication, reduce hot flushes and night sweats, and help with insomnia. If your symptoms are severe, you may decide that the benefits outweigh the risks. If you are one of the few apple-shaped women who experience low-oestrogen symptoms, listen to your body. You may actually benefit from low doses of HT. Ideally, you should have a good doctor-patient partnership that allows you to discuss these types of issues in detail, and to make health-related decisions together.

The only form of HT I would generally recommend for apple-shaped women who feel they must have hormones is a transdermal oestradiol patch, such as Evorel or Estraderm. The patch is thin, transparent and tiny – only about 1cm (½in) in diameter – so it is barely noticeable. It doesn't come off in the bath or shower, or even during vigorous physical activity. It comes in several dosages, and I usually like to start my patients with the lowest, 0.025 milligrams, and increase it if necessary. This low dose preserves bone density, reduces hot flushes, helps improve sleep and treats or prevents vaginal dryness and atrophy.

Apple-shaped women who have not had a hysterectomy and are considering using either of these products also need to take progesterone to reduce the risk of endometrial cancer. That's because apple-shaped women are likely to have more unopposed oestrogen as they go into menopause, which means that they probably have a uterine lining build-up that needs to be shed. I recommend a 12-day course of natural progesterone (Prometrium, 200 milligrams daily, or crinone gel) to balance out the remaining oestrogen. At the end of the 12 days, women will usually get a period, so the final uterine lining is cleaned out. Now, they are starting with a clean slate, so to speak. If they then decide to go on HT, they are less likely to have erratic or heavy bleeding, and they've taken another step towards preventing endometrial cancer.

Again, I *do not recommend oral oestrogen to apple-shaped women.* But if it is absolutely necessary, they should only take the lowest dose of either Climaval (oestradiol, 0.5 milligrams, available by taking half of a 1 milligram tablet) or Premarin (conjugated oestrogen, 0.325 milligrams). They should definitely *not* take Provera (conjugated oestrogen with medroxyprogesterone), which contains a more potent androgenic progestin, and was shown in the Women's Health Initiative study to increase heart disease risk.

HT Recommendations for Pear-Shaped Women

If you are a pear-shaped woman and would like to try HT, I won't talk you out of it. Thin pear-shaped women derive the greatest benefit and often do very well on HT. For example, one woman I treated, Denise, was very thin – a skinny pear – and therefore had a high risk of osteoporosis. Her bone density was already on the low side, and as with all women, it would only get worse as she got older. She went on HT, and her body sucked it up. It was as though she were a sponge for oestrogen. She didn't even bleed! No matter how much she took, it did not cause the types of uncomfortable physical changes that I'd seen in my apple-shaped patients. Her breasts stayed normal, her body shape didn't change, she didn't become bloated and her sense of herself remained exactly the same as it was before she took the hormones. In fact, she said she felt more like her usual self after receiving the oestrogen treatment. She did great, and I know that she's still perfectly healthy today. She gradually lowered the dose over the years and is now deciding whether to stop altogether. She plans to let her body decide whether she needs to continue taking hormones or not. I've seen that over and over in my pear-shaped patients, and that's my recommendation for pear-shaped readers, too: let your body tell you what is right for *you*.

There are many reasons why HT is a viable option for pear-shaped women:

◆ HT has been shown to prevent women from adding visceral fat, therefore it helps pear-shaped women avoid becoming apple-shaped after menopause.

◆ Oestrogen helps increase bone density and muscle mass, which may help prevent osteoporosis.

◆ Oral oestrogens actually can improve some cardiovascular risk factors. Although they raise triglycerides, lower insulin sensitivity, and increase levels of the inflammation marker CRP (all bad for the heart), oestrogens also have been shown to raise HDL cholesterol, lower total cholesterol and reduce the amount of weight naturally gained during and after menopause (all good for the heart). Because pear-shaped women have many fewer risk factors for heart disease, the bad HT effects shouldn't be enough to push them over the edge into disease, and the good HT effects may keep them healthier longer.

◆ Oestrogen may be protective against dementia, although the data are confusing. Many scientists and physicians believe that if oestrogen is started early in menopause, it may stave off Alzheimer's disease. But oestrogen given later in life may increase the risk.

Pear-shaped women can safely take most forms of oestrogen, but I still think it's a good idea to take the minimum amount needed to control your menopausal symptoms. I typically recommend the transdermal patch Evorel or Estraderm (oestradiol, 0.025 to 0.05 milligrams; see the description for apple-shaped women on page 70), or pills – Premarin (conjugated oestrogen, 0.3 to 0.625 milligrams) or Estrace (oestradiol, 0.5 to 1.0 milligrams). Women with a uterus will need to add progesterone to protect against endometrial cancer. I recommend natural progesterone in the form of vaginal gel (Crinone), which is taken for 12 days every one to three months depending on the dose of oestrogen. When you stop taking it, you may shed your uterine lining if you have a sufficient build-up; but often women on the lowest oestrogen dose will either spot or not bleed at all.

There is also the Nuvelle, a transdermal patch that contains both oestrogen (0.05 milligrams of oestradiol) and progesterone/ norethindrone. Some women may find this more convenient than taking pills, and it seems to be well tolerated.

ALTERNATIVES TO HORMONES FOR MENOPAUSAL AND PERIMENOPAUSAL WOMEN

Nobody *has* to take hormones for relief of menopause symptoms. Every woman will have different symptoms with different levels of severity. One woman's minor inconvenience will be another woman's version of a living hell. Your choice will depend on how uncomfortable you are, what your personal family health history is and what risks you are willing to take. Regardless of whether you take hormones or not, 75 per cent of all women have no further symptoms five years after menopause. Some women stop having symptoms within two years. So waiting it out is always an option.

Other options include some of the complementary or alternative medicine options that are becoming increasingly popular. But popularity doesn't equal effectiveness. Researchers have found that dong quai, evening primrose oil, ginseng, red clover, wild yam cream and vitamin E are no better at relieving women's menopause symptoms than sugar pills. In fact, one common alternative treatment, oil of chaste tree berry (*Vitex agnus-castus*), was found to actually increase the number of hot flushes and night sweats in some women, and the most common side effect was depression. Kava (*Piper methysticum*) has been shown to cause liver problems in some people. I cannot recommend any of these alternative treatments.

Only two alternative remedies have been scientifically shown to have any effect on symptoms of menopause: black cohosh and soya foods.

◆ **Black cohosh.** This herb, also known as *Actaea racemosa,* has been used by healers to treat gynaecologic and other health conditions for hundreds of years. Most scientific research has shown that taking the standardised product Remifemin (its only active ingredient is black cohosh) reduced the frequency and intensity of hot flushes significantly, but no one knows exactly how or why it works. The biologically active ingredients have not been isolated yet. However, the fact that it works means that it has some powerful actions in the body. Because no study has looked at the long-term effects of taking black cohosh, the American College of Obstetrics and Gynecology approved its use for up to six months only. Some concern has been raised about its safety, especially by scientists who have suggested that black cohosh may cause liver failure in some women, and may spur the spread of breast cancer in women who already have the disease. I'm not convinced that we know everything we need to know about the safety of black cohosh, and I would be reluctant to recommend it right now. Please talk with your physician before starting to use it.

◆ **Soya foods.** My favourite hormone alternative is soya foods, which can provide relief of mild menopausal symptoms. I particularly recommend it for apple-shaped women who cannot or should not take HT. Soya foods contain compounds called *phytooestrogens,* which basically means 'oestrogens from plants'. These compounds include isoflavones, lignans and coumestans – words that sound unfamiliar now, but trust me . . . you'll be hearing more about them in the future as research continues. Phytooestrogens can have a similar effect to the weak, 'diluted' oestrone produced by pear-shaped women. Some studies have shown that these compounds help reduce the severity and frequency of hot flushes, but the results are not consistent. There is also some preliminary and observational evidence that soya may also help protect some women against heart disease and breast cancer – which is of particular importance to apple-shaped women because they have a higher risk of both diseases.

It is extremely important to note, however, that known benefits of soya are limited to natural phytochemicals found in foods. There are supplements available that contain higher concentrations of isoflavones, the supposed active component of soya foods, but this is one of those times when *more* is not necessarily *better.* No one knows what effects high levels of isoflavones might have. Just as very high levels of natural oestrogen in our bodies can increase our risk of disease, higher levels of plant oestrogens may also be harmful. In fact, there is some evidence that soya supplements – as opposed to soya from foods – may *increase* the risk of breast cancer. I recommend soya foods to all my patients, but I *highly* recommend them to my apple-shaped patients. (See chapter 11 for more information about soya foods and specific recommendations.)

In mainstream medicine, researchers have discovered that some women can get relief from menopausal symptoms by taking certain antidepressants. The best antidepressants for menopause are Efexor (venlafaxine) and Seroxat (paroxetine). Along with improving mood, these medications can also reduce hot flushes and improve sleep. (Not all antidepressants will help with hot flushes and other symptoms.) If you are having considerable discomfort, talk with your health care provider about whether you might be a good candidate for this type of treatment.

MAKING THE HORMONE DECISION

In the end, making the decision about whether to take hormones at any point in your life is a balancing act. You have to evaluate carefully the risks versus the benefits. Look at your family history. If you have relatives who have had breast cancer, you might want to avoid both birth control pills and HT. But if osteoporosis runs in your family, you'll have to decide if taking HT and thereby avoiding debilitating bone disease is worth the possible increase in breast cancer risk.

If you are thinking of starting HT, remember that there are side effects to every medication. Make sure you fully understand what will happen. I knew a woman who was astonished to learn that her periods might start up again when she began hormones. Talk with your health care practitioner until all your questions and concerns are answered. Make sure you understand what body sensations are normal and what dangerous side effects to guard against. These may be different depending on the exact hormone preparation used. Ultimately, the decision is yours . . . based on sound medical information and professional guidance.

Action Items for Chapter 4: The Hormone Question

Every woman aged 30 and older should take some time to size up her health. Women of all ages need baseline health numbers to use for comparison in the coming years. Those who are currently taking HT or considering starting will have special testing needs to determine whether they have any disease risk factors that will make HT hazardous to their health. At your next health check, talk with your doctor about the following tests:

◆ A complete fasting blood lipid profile (to look especially at HDL and triglyceride levels).

◆ Blood pressure.

◆ CRP levels measured by a blood test.

◆ A gynaecology exam. This will include a smear test to look for precancerous changes to the cervix, a test for human papillomavirus (HPV) for women age 30 and older, a pelvic exam and a breast exam.

◆ Record test results on the Body Shape Health Log for your shape (on pages 328 and 329) in the appropriate columns.

◆ Repeat these measurements as often as you and your doctor decide is necessary. Record all new test results on your Body Shape Health Log. Comparing the initial numbers to the follow-up numbers – and to your target goal – will help you to monitor your response to the hormones and help you and your doctor decide if it is safe to continue taking them.

◆ If you take hormones – before or after menopause – keep a brief journal to record your symptoms or side effects. For example, record instances of nausea, breast tenderness, bloating, headaches, hot flushes, night sweats or any other problem. You can also track the days when you bleed, and make a brief note about how heavy or light the flow is. This will be valuable information to help your health care provider adjust your dosage so you can feel your best. Record your good responses to treatment, too, such as improved sleep, fewer hot flushes, less vaginal dryness, et cetera.

Take to Heart . . .

◆ Your peace of mind is of utmost importance. If the risks involved with taking hormones scare you too much, don't take them. There are alternative birth control methods, including the use of condoms, diaphragms with spermicidal jelly, intrauterine devices (IUD) and tubal ligation. (The 'rhythm method' or other unprotected practices do not work well at all and cannot be recommended.) There are also plenty of options for treatment of menopausal symptoms. Discuss your concerns with your doctor and don't make any decisions until you feel confident.

◆ You are not locked into any decision. If you decide to try hormones but later find you can't tolerate the side effects, you can always stop or change the type and/or dose. You don't have to continue down the same road for the rest of your life.

CHAPTER 5

The Metabolic Syndrome and Type 2 Diabetes

Until complications set in, the metabolic syndrome and type 2 diabetes get very little respect from anyone, mainly because these disorders are so poorly understood. It's no wonder. The metabolic syndrome and type 2 diabetes are difficult to visualise because there are no outward, physical signs that allow us to see the course of the disease. They don't arouse much worry because they don't cause immediate pain or discomfort. They are not caused by a virus or bacterium, so our usual methods of understanding disease don't work here. Plus, the underlying medical concepts are so intertwined, so convoluted and so mysterious that even scientists are still trying to figure out all the various physiologic connections.

The metabolic syndrome (sometimes called syndrome X, or the metabolic syndrome X) and diabetes are both disorders in the way our bodies use food for energy. The normal processes that allow glucose from the foods we eat to leave the bloodstream, enter cells and provide fuel for the body no longer work the way that they should. Early in the disease process, there are no symptoms, nothing to alert an individual that she might have a problem. Simple blood tests can easily detect the metabolic syndrome or type 2 diabetes at their very early stages, before they have a chance to cause permanent damage or even death. And it is becoming increasingly clear that one of the most potent warning signs of possible disease is having an apple shape.

Tragically, many general practitioners dismiss some of the early warning signs of these diseases. Doctors are taught to check for high cholesterol, but there has traditionally been much less emphasis on some of the other hallmarks of the metabolic syndrome – triglycerides, high-density lipoprotein (HDL) cholesterol or borderline abnormal blood sugar. And there has been no attention paid to the role of body shape, how *apple-shaped women have an increased risk of these metabolic disorders, regardless of their body weight.* Perhaps doctors don't know about the apple-shaped connection, don't bother to measure waist circumference or don't have the time to explain the intricacies of what is going on in a woman's body. But the outcome is the same: too many women go on to develop the metabolic syndrome and diabetes and never receive any information about how to prevent them. And women, who generally rely on their physicians for medical information, often don't have the knowledge or the confidence to ask.

What's worse is that even when a diagnosis is made, most people – patients and physicians alike – respond with only lukewarm concern. Despite the seriousness of these disorders, studies repeatedly show that only about one-third of people with diabetes reach their target goals for blood glucose, blood pressure and cholesterol. This means that they are not controlling their disease; rather, their disease is controlling them. Can you imagine this same lack of concern applied to other illnesses, such as the flu, stomach ulcers or cancer? Hardly. So why do people routinely ignore the risks associated with the metabolic syndrome and diabetes?

Studies repeatedly show that only about one-third of
people with diabetes reach their target goals for blood
glucose, blood pressure and cholesterol.

I believe that part of the general apathy comes from the language we use to discuss the metabolic syndrome and type 2 diabetes. Those names are not descriptive enough. They don't tell us what is going on in the body. They don't convey a sense of urgency for treatment or any notion of exactly how debilitating these disorders can be. People with diabetes talk about having 'high blood sugar' or 'a touch of sugar', which sounds like something that could happen if you eat a couple of Mars Bars. In reality, that 'high blood sugar' is a common cause of blindness, amputations, coma and death. That's why I think these disorders need a public relations makeover. A few years ago, the American Heart Association decided that the public didn't properly appreciate the seriousness of strokes, and so they began calling them 'brain attacks' – heart attacks in the head. It seems to be working. More people now know the signs of a brain attack, which means that they can seek treatment earlier. I think the time has come to rename the metabolic syndrome and type 2 diabetes, to give them catchier, more descriptive nicknames to grab our attention. If it were up to me, I'd call the metabolic syndrome *'silent killer disorder'*, and I'd call type 2 diabetes *'body deterioration disease'*.

Does that grab your attention?

These disorders are the shark in the water – hidden, sneaky and deadly. You'll see signs if you look carefully, but if you ignore them, they'll bite. Hard. And it can be very difficult to shake them loose. The key phrase, of course, is 'if you ignore them'. As serious as the metabolic syndrome and type 2 diabetes are, they are also among the most controllable of physical ailments. It is totally within our power to either prevent or manage these disorders and live normal, healthy lives. Being diagnosed with the metabolic syndrome or diabetes is not an automatic death sentence. It is possible to swim with the sharks without being bitten. In fact, I'd say that getting diagnosed is lucky, and the earlier the better. Too often doctors miss the subtle blood abnormalities that signal the early start of these diseases, or they may not check for them at all. Isn't it better to know that the disease is there so you can take steps to control or reverse it, than to be surprised to learn that a disease you didn't know you had has already caused irreversible damage?

METABOLISM BASICS

Your body is a complex, interconnected weaving of blood vessels, nerves, body tissue, hormones, organs and other critical parts. Each part is made up of living cells that need fuel in order to survive. Without the right kinds and amounts of fuel, everything will eventually shut down. Slowly but surely, piece by piece, our bodies will stop working. Cells will die. Blood vessels will close down. Organs will fail. Everything deteriorates. If you are diagnosed with the disease early enough, you can prevent it all. But if you wait, some of the damage will be beyond repair.

When we are healthy, the food we eat is broken down into its component parts – proteins, fats and carbohydrates. These are further broken down into smaller molecules that serve specific functions in the body. Carbohydrates are broken down into simple sugars, mainly glucose. All of our cells use glucose for energy; it is the fuel that powers our bodies. But cells are like little fortresses. They are surrounded by a thick wall called a membrane, which regulates what comes in and what goes out by a complex system of locks, codes, pumps and chaperones. Without a key to open a lock or the exact coded combination, the cell will stay sealed up and secure.

After we eat a meal, glucose from carbohydrates enters the blood-stream and circulates throughout the body. (Testing for *blood glucose* tells you how much glucose or sugar is circulating in your body at a particular time.) The rise in blood glucose signals the pancreas to release the hormone *insulin,* which fits like a key into the insulin receptors – which we can think of as the imaginary locks in the cell membrane. Glucose molecules leave the bloodstream and enter the cells within seconds of when insulin connects with receptors in the membranes. As blood glucose levels drop, the pancreas stops releasing insulin and the body waits for its next meal.

Type 2 Diabetes

That's what happens when everything is functioning properly, a normal metabolic state. But what happens if something goes wrong? Imagine, for example, how the sequence of events changes if there is a problem with insulin, which occurs in type 1 or type 2 diabetes. *Type 1 diabetes* is the result of an autoimmune reaction in which the insulin-producing beta cells of the pancreas are destroyed. Because insulin can no longer be produced, it cannot be released in response to a rise in blood glucose. Without the insulin key, the membrane stays closed and glucose cannot enter the cells; and without glucose, the cells eventually die and the body fails. That's why all people who have type 1 diabetes need to take insulin, usually by injection. Only about 10 per cent of all diabetes cases are type 1 diabetes, and it almost always occurs before age 20.

In *type 2 diabetes,* the pancreas starts out healthy. After a meal, when blood glucose levels rise, the pancreas releases plenty of insulin. The problem is that the insulin is no longer capable of opening all the membrane doors. It's as if some of the locks have been changed so that the key doesn't fit anymore. At this point, we say that the cells have become *insulin resistant.* Glucose doesn't enter the cells as easily as it used to, and some of the cells starve. Because blood glucose levels remain high, the pancreas continues to pump out insulin to try to compensate. Having too much insulin in the blood is called *hyperinsulinaemia,* and in most cases it goes hand in hand with insulin resistance. Eventually, the beta cells of the pancreas can't keep up with the insulin demand and the pancreas stops making insulin altogether, a state called *insulin exhaustion.* Over time, cells become more and more insulin resistant – more and more imaginary locks get changed – until very little glucose enters the cells. If glucose can't enter the cells, it stays in the bloodstream, leading to high levels of measured blood glucose (*hyperglycaemia*).

It isn't just a question of either being healthy *or* having diabetes. There is a continuum of disease, from healthy insulin functioning on one end, to full-fledged diabetes on the other end, with a range of unhealthy insulin resistance in the middle ground.

At a certain point, insulin resistance leads to persistently high blood glucose, even after an overnight fast. That is diabetes. Healthy people generally maintain a steady blood glucose level of between 60 and 99 mg/dL. (We always have some glucose in our bloodstream because our brains need a constant supply of energy.) To test for diabetes, the doctor will test your blood after a night of fasting. A fasting blood glucose of 99 mg/dL or lower is considered normal. If blood glucose levels are between 100 and 125 mg/dL, that is called *impaired glucose tolerance* or *prediabetes.* Fasting blood glucose levels 126 mg/dL or higher are diagnosed as type 2 diabetes. So you see, it isn't just a question of either being healthy *or* having diabetes. There is a continuum of disease, from healthy insulin functioning on one end, to full-fledged diabetes on the other end, with a range of unhealthy insulin resistance in the middle ground.

The Metabolic Syndrome

The metabolic syndrome isn't a disease so much as a description of a cluster of physiological problems that add up to a very high risk of diabetes and heart disease (hence my nickname, *silent killer disorder*). To receive a diagnosis of the metabolic syndrome, you must have at least three of the following:

◆ high blood glucose after fasting (≥ 100 mg/dL)

◆ high waist circumference (> 90cm (35½in) for women; > 100cm (39½in) for men)

◆ hypertension (blood pressure ≥ 130/85 mm Hg)

◆ high triglycerides after fasting (≥ 150 mg/dL)

◆ low levels of high-density lipoprotein (HDL) cholesterol (< 50 mg/dL for women; < 40 mg/dL for men)

Each of these measurements is a sign that something is going wrong in the body. The concept of the metabolic syndrome was developed when scientists discovered that a combination of three or more of these signs make a perfect recipe for heart disease.

The metabolic syndrome is also a warning sign that type 2 diabetes is lurking about. In fact, about 40 per cent of patients with impaired glucose tolerance develop diabetes within 5 to 10 years; the rest either remain with lower insulin sensitivity, or they can regain normal metabolic function after making appropriate lifestyle changes (and sometimes with the help of insulin-sensitising medications). The tricky thing about the metabolic disorder is that you'll never know you have it unless you go to the doctor and have fasting blood tests done. So tens of millions of people are on the road to developing diabetes, but they don't know it. And once diabetes develops, it has been estimated that about 10 years go by before the disease is diagnosed. That's enough time for 15 to 20 per cent of patients to start to go blind from diabetic retinopathy (when the delicate blood vessels to the eye are destroyed), and for about 10 per cent to have the beginnings of kidney failure.

Millie's Diabetes Story

My sister Millie is a prime example of what happens when a woman doesn't get all the information she needs to stay healthy. She is an educated, intelligent woman, but she went from having the metabolic syndrome to having diabetes without ever knowing that there was a problem. It started with weight gain. I don't normally treat family members, but several years ago, I was desperate to help her. She had gained a lot of weight – much of it around her waist – and I was worried about her health. Before recommending a diet, I did comprehensive blood work. She had nonfasting blood glucose levels that were mildly high – about 116. Without doing a fasting glucose test, it was impossible to know what was going on, so I recommended that she see her family doctor. He did the fasting glucose test, and told her she was fine.

In truth, she wasn't fine. She had prediabetes. Unfortunately, she didn't learn about it until years later, after she got a hold of her old medical records and after she understood how to read the test result numbers. It was also after she was diagnosed with diabetes at a routine physical examination. By then her blood glucose levels were dangerously high, and yet she had no symptoms – the silent killer had struck again. If she hadn't had that routine exam, the disease would have gone undiagnosed for years – possibly leading to an early death from heart attack. Today, Millie admits that she didn't take the diagnosis seriously at first. She thought that it was just a sign that she needed to avoid sugar and lose weight, and that she would be fine once she got motivated. The problem is that diabetes causes small blood vessels to become damaged. Over years, blood flow to certain body parts becomes hindered. Nerves can die. Eyes fail. Limbs can become gangrenous and require amputation.

Millie didn't get scared until she developed painful neuropathy in her feet. That got her attention. Now, she's a model of control. She owns a blood glucose measuring device called a glucometer to monitor her blood sugar regularly; she knows her target goals for glucose, cholesterol and blood pressure; and she actively looks for diet and lifestyle changes to help control her weight. It took a permanent and potentially limb-threatening problem to make her understand the seriousness of diabetes. I honestly believe that if she had known that her apple-shaped body predisposed her to insulin resistance – that it wasn't all her fault – then she would have not felt so guilty and remained in denial for so long.

BODY SHAPE AND METABOLIC DISORDERS

Exactly what causes the metabolic syndrome and diabetes is still a mystery, but we can identify a few of the factors that make some people more susceptible to the disease than others. Part of the risk is genetic – you can inherit a predisposition for the disease from your parents and grandparents. But the number one cause of these metabolic problems is obesity. The link between diabetes and obesity is so strong that some scientists have suggested calling the disease 'diabesity'. There are several theories about how obesity is related to these metabolic disorders. One thought is that the chemical changes caused by excess fat somehow alter the cells' insulin receptors so that the insulin key can no longer fit. When excess weight is lost, the insulin receptors resume their original configuration, and insulin sensitivity increases. Other theories centre around the complex interactions of body hormones and their regulation. Some researchers have even asked the next obvious question: Is it all fat that contributes to the risk of diabetes, or just visceral fat?

The link between diabetes and obesity
is so strong that some scientists have suggested
calling the disease 'diabesity'.

It turns out that visceral fat is, indeed, the diabetes-causing culprit. Scientists believe that the metabolically active visceral fat causes too many free fatty acids to be dumped into the bloodstream (via the liver), which can cause glucose intolerance and insulin resistance. So having large amounts of visceral fat can wreak hormonal havoc – women with the metabolic syndrome may be pushed further along the insulin resistance continuum into diabetes, and those with diabetes will find it more difficult to regain control over blood glucose levels. Women who have a large waist circumference *and* high triglycerides – a combination I call the 'triglyceride waist' – are at imminent risk of developing the metabolic syndrome or even diabetes. An American study conducted by researchers at the Centers for Disease Control and Prevention (CDC) showed that people with a triglyceride waist were three times more likely to have diabetes than people without a triglyceride waist.

As powerful a predictor as the triglyceride waist is, the test for triglycerides is a nuisance that requires a 12-hour fast and blood work. Which makes you think: wouldn't it be nice if there was some other measure, some alternate way of deciding who was most at risk so that they could get further testing? Well, there is. And, of course, I'm talking about body shape.

Having an apple shape is a risk factor for developing metabolic disorders, and apple-shaped women with a waist circumference greater than 90cm (35½in) should be considered at high risk and tested immediately. In 2003, researchers in Australia conducted a study of more than 11,000 men and women. They discovered that *body shape was the strongest predictor of future diabetes,* stronger than either body mass index (BMI) or waist circumference. Women who had an apple-shaped figure were more likely to develop diabetes, as well as high blood pressure, high triglycerides and low HDL cholesterol – all the risk factors for the metabolic syndrome. And the larger the WHR, and the larger the waist circumference, the higher the risk. For apple-shaped women, the risk for the metabolic syndrome and type 2 diabetes is high, and it gets higher for every additional centimetre around their waists.

Women with polycystic ovary syndrome (PCOS), that extreme of the apple-shaped physiology, have the highest risks. Comparisons have shown that 46 per cent of women with PCOS have the metabolic syndrome, compared with about 23 per cent of women without PCOS – double the average rate. But like everyone else, women with PCOS can stop the progression to diabetes and even reverse the metabolic slide by reducing their waist circumference and, in some instances, by taking medication (see below).

Pear-shaped women seem to be somehow protected from diabetes and the metabolic syndrome by their pear-zone fat, which doesn't contribute to free fatty acids in the bloodstream and therefore doesn't contribute to insulin resistance. One fascinating study compared postmenopausal women who were overweight but still had high insulin sensitivity (classified as 'metabolically normal') with similarly overweight women who had low insulin sensitivity (classified as 'metabolically abnormal' or insulin resistant). They all had an average BMI of 31.5, and their average weight was about 85kg (13 stone, 5lb). The researchers found that the women who were classified as metabolically normal had *half the amount of visceral fat* as the women classified as metabolically abnormal – even though they had the same total amount of body fat.

Other research has shown that having a large hip and/or thigh circumference equates to about a 40 per cent *decrease* in the risk for developing diabetes. Another study found that overweight post-menopausal women with diabetes tend to have less lower-body fat (pear-zone fat) than similarly overweight women without diabetes. The

Nurses' Health Study did a direct comparison, and the researchers found that the risk of developing diabetes was three times higher in apple-shaped women than in pear-shaped women.

Unfortunately, this diabetes-prone effect of an apple shape extends to women who are not overweight. It has been estimated that about 18 per cent of women with low insulin sensitivity have a normal body weight and fall into the 'ideal' category for body mass index. One study looked specifically at a group of these women and found that they had a greater per centage of body fat, and a greater amount of visceral fat than women who had normal insulin sensitivity. In other words, even apple-shaped women who have relatively low body weight have an increased risk of developing the metabolic syndrome. But please remember, this increased risk does not have to be your destiny. These disorders are highly preventable.

THE DIABETES EFFECTS OF MEDICATIONS

Any medication that causes weight gain will automatically lead to an increased risk of metabolic disorders. The worst offenders are the class of drugs called glucocorticoids (commonly referred to as 'steroids'), such as betamethasone dexamethasone, hydrocortisone, methylprednisolone, prednisolone or prednisone. These medications are used to treat a variety of inflammation-related problems, but their actions lead to weight gain and cause the liver to release more glucose into the bloodstream. They also tend to increase visceral fat, and they independently increase insulin resistance, although the extent of the increase depends on the specific type and dosage of medication used. For example, after less than a week of glucocorticoids treatment, one study showed that dexamethasone treatment caused a 30 per cent drop in insulin sensitivity; whereas another study found a 64 per cent drop with prednisone treatment. Although the body compensates for these changes in the short term, long-term use of these medications can lead to diabetes, especially in people who are already showing signs of metabolic problems. Women who need to take steroids long term can develop something called Cushing's syndrome, which causes them to develop an apple body shape, along with additional symptoms of thin skin susceptible to bruising and excess body fat in their neck and upper back.

Although all women need to be aware of the increased visceral fat and insulin resistance effects of glucocorticoids medications, this is especially true for apple-shaped women who already have a tendency to have visceral fat and insulin resistance. I have had apple-shaped patients who had to take steroids and unsuspectingly developed diabetes, which then went away once they stopped taking the medication. And I have also noticed that apple-shaped women seem to become even more apple-shaped with steroids. Short-term use of steroids, such as for poison ivy or allergies, is usually potent but quick – a one-week treatment – and it shouldn't do any long-term damage. If you need steroids long term for serious conditions such as Crohn's disease or asthma, then work with your doctor to figure out the lowest possible dose to keep the disease under control.

Apple-shaped women, who already have a high risk of diabetes, need to have their blood sugars monitored regularly if they need to take glucocorticoids. If they already have some signs of insulin resistance, it is entirely possible that blood glucose levels may rise into the diabetic range, and therefore they may need to take medication for diabetes, too. Apple-shaped women will also need to exercise and watch their diets even more closely to avoid putting on too much more visceral fat. Because steroids also increase bone turnover and bone resorption, they can cause osteoporosis, especially of the spine. Pear-shaped women will need to be more concerned with osteoporosis and should consider hormone therapy after menopause to offset some of the bone loss due to steroid medication. All women on long-term steroids will need to have yearly bone density scans, and should take calcium and vitamin D supplements.

Another group of drugs that apple-shaped women need to be careful of are generally called atypical antipsychotic medications. Don't let the name bother you – these drugs are also commonly prescribed to people who have trouble sleeping or are in chronic pain. Some of these medications have been shown to increase the risk of type 2 diabetes, increase blood lipids, and cause weight gain – particularly around the waist. The most commonly prescribed drugs that have been shown to cause this effect are Clozaril (clozapine), Risperdal (risperidone), Seroquel (quetiapine) and Zyprexa (olanzapine). Apple-shaped women who are taking these medications should talk with their physicians to see if they can be switched to a different medication, or to have their blood glucose levels and blood lipid levels tested to monitor for diabetes or risk factors for heart disease. If you are taking one of these medications, do not stop taking it without the advice and consent of your prescribing physician.

PREVENTION OF DIABETES AND THE METABOLIC SYNDROME

Smoking

If you smoke, stop. Studies have shown that smoking independently increases the risk of developing diabetes by between 40 and 100 per cent. Smoking also seems to increase the amount of visceral fat gained, so it increases risk on two separate fronts. Apple-shaped women who smoke, whether they are overweight or lean, are virtually signing up in advance for diabetes and a heart attack. The only time I have seen heart attacks in women before menopause is if they either smoked or had the metabolic syndrome or diabetes. Even if you've tried to quit before, I urge you to try again. There are many new stop-smoking products on the market, and your doctor can help guide you to the method that might work best for you. This will be the most difficult, and yet most important, health step you ever take.

If you smoke, stop. Studies have shown that smoking
independently increases the risk of developing diabetes
by between 40 and 100 per cent.

Diet and Exercise

Follow the programmes in this book. The programme for apple-shaped women is designed for total health, including diabetes prevention. Studies have shown that you can decrease your risk of developing diabetes by up to 60 per cent by diet and exercise alone. This is true for men and women of all ages and from all ethnic groups. By working on health by centimetres, instead of weight, and following the programme in Part 3, I estimate that most apple-shaped women can cut their risk of diabetes in half.

You can decrease your risk of developing diabetes by
up to 60 per cent by diet and exercise alone.

Medication

If lifestyle changes aren't a realistic option right now, or if those changes haven't worked for you, the second line of attack might be medication. Some drugs are useful for staving off diabetes in people with the metabolic syndrome. The most commonly used is metformin (Glucophage). It works to improve insulin action, reduce your appetite and lower blood glucose. One study showed that, used on its own, metformin can decrease the number of people who develop diabetes by about 25 per cent. This medication commonly causes some weight loss, and therefore it is a good choice for apple-shaped women with the metabolic syndrome or diabetes who need additional help losing weight to keep their disease under control. It can cause mild gastrointestinal upset or nausea, but it is mild and not serious, and can even help women lose weight because of their decreased interest in food.

Another commonly used drug is Avandia (rosiglitazone), which also lowers glucose levels. Rosiglitazone acts as an insulin sensitiser – it allows the insulin to work better at the level of the cell (like helping the insulin key work in a less-than-perfect lock). Rosiglitazone can cause weight gain – but mainly in the pear zone. Its main effects are that it improves blood glucose control and blood lipid profiles by lowering triglycerides and LDL cholesterol and by raising HDL cholesterol. It also causes very few side effects. The only significant problem is the possibility of fluid retention, so it is never given to people with heart failure.

Precose (acarbose) is sometimes prescribed to people with diabetes to help them regain control over their blood glucose, and it is being tested as a possible diabetes preventive in people with the metabolic syndrome. Acarbose delays the absorption of carbohydrates from the small intestine, thereby reducing high blood glucose after meals. In addition, it lowers blood pressure, improves blood lipids levels, shrinks waist circumference, and reduces the risk of heart attack by more than 60 per cent.

Xenical (orlistat) is a weight-loss medication that offers the additional benefit of a reduced risk of diabetes. Studies have shown that people with the metabolic syndrome who change their diet, start to exercise and take orlistat are about one-third less likely to develop type 2 diabetes. They also lost about 50 per cent more weight than people who did not take the medication. Orlistat works by blocking the absorption of fat from the intestines. This means that women who take this medication must be *very* careful with their diets. There's no room for 'cheating'. If you eat fatty foods while taking orlistat, the result is what is euphemistically called 'anal leakage', which can happen unexpectedly and can be extremely embarrassing. If you are an overweight apple-shaped woman – with or without diabetes or the metabolic syndrome – and you are having trouble reducing your waist despite being diligent about controlling your diet, consider talking with your doctor about orlistat.

DIABETES IS NOT INEVITABLE

The metabolic syndrome and type 2 diabetes are so common today that they are often assumed to be just another age-related cross to bear. If you have an apple shape and mildly high blood glucose levels, both you and your doctor may be fooled into thinking you are okay. You are not. These diseases are partially genetic, but predominantly related to visceral fat. For most people, type 2 diabetes is entirely preventable.

You don't have to become sick
as you grow older.

Action Items for Chapter 5:
The Metabolic Syndrome and Type 2 Diabetes

◆ All apple-shaped women should have certain tests by the time they turn 40 – a fasting glucose test, a fasting lipid panel (triglycerides, HDL and LDL, and total cholesterol), and a blood pressure measurement. (If you are an apple-shaped woman over age 40 who has never been tested, call your doctor for these tests immediately.) If your tests are normal, repeat them every two to three years, or with every two or three centimetres you gain around your waist. Record all numbers on your Body Shape Health Log (these begin on page 328).

◆ If you have diabetes, become an expert in your disease. Ask for pamphlets, visit a diabetes care specialist, visit reliable websites that provide accurate information, or contact Diabetes UK (www.diabetes.org.uk) for information.

◆ If you are apple-shaped and are pregnant or thinking about becoming pregnant, talk to your doctor about being tested for diabetes. Many women are routinely checked for diabetes during the second trimester of pregnancy, but you may need to be tested earlier. If you are overweight, apple-shaped and/or have a family history of diabetes, I recommend getting tested for diabetes before pregnancy (if you are thinking about becoming pregnant), or at the beginning of your second trimester (if you are already pregnant). Pregnancy can cause a temporary form of diabetes called *gestational diabetes,* which requires special treatment.

◆ Review your pregnancy history. If you had gestational diabetes during any of your previous pregnancies, you are much more likely to develop full-blown diabetes in the future. Following the pro-gramme here can help prevent you from developing full-blown diabetes, but you need to be even more vigilant than most.

◆ Get enough sleep. One study found that being sleep deprived for less than a week (sleeping four hours per night for six nights) lowered glucose tolerance. I know sleeplessness seems to be a given in today's hectic society. We all have too much to do, and not enough hours to do it in. Don't let sleep be the part of your life that suffers – doctor's orders!

◆ Read the next chapter on heart disease. If you've noticed, the words 'heart attack' and 'heart disease' appear frequently in this chapter. Most women with the metabolic syndrome or diabetes don't realise how much their life depends on understanding heart-related risks. Even if you don't think heart disease is important to you now, it is important to understand the connections.

Take to Heart...

◆ Think small. Sometimes even minor changes can have unexpectedly powerful results. We are so used to thinking in terms of 'dropping two dress sizes' or 'losing 20 pounds by Friday' that we start to believe that we must see big changes fast. In the long run, that kind of expectation will limit your success. Focus on the small changes that will make the biggest difference in your life. The women who cut their risk of diabetes in half by following diet and exercise recommendations lost an average of *only 5cm (2in) off their waists.* That was enough to help delay or prevent diabetes.

◆ Think *control.* Ultimately, your health is not up to your mother, your husband, your partner or your doctor. It is up to you. Throughout the book, I explain how to take control of your health information, your body, your test results, your medications and other health aspects. But you have to be ready to hear it. Above all else, diabetes is a disease of control. The sooner you are ready to take action, the healthier you'll be.

◆ Denial and guilt are the biggest challenges for apple-shaped women who are overweight apples. Society vilifies women for their body shape. So do many physicians. Women may be made to feel that diabetes is their fault, when really they have this visceral fat predisposition. The more they try to lose weight, the guiltier they feel and the greater the denial of physical problems. After all, having an 'obesity-related' disease would be another sign of failure to women who have difficulty losing weight. Prevention and control are entirely possible, if you choose to think positively. Disease is not a failure. Ignoring it won't make it go away.

CHAPTER 6

Heart Disease, Stroke and Inflammation

When I was just beginning this book, my writing colleague's 74-year-old mother-in-law, Ginny, died of a sudden, massive heart attack. She had awakened in the middle of the night feeling sweaty and nauseated and found that she was having some difficulty breathing. No crushing chest pain. No shooting pain down the left arm. None of the classic symptoms we've all memorised. She cried out for help, and family members rushed to call the paramedics. She died before reaching the hospital.

Ginny was a classic apple-shaped woman, with very thin legs and a large waist. She smoked moderately, a few cigarettes a day, but she was trying to quit because she was afraid of getting lung cancer. She joked about her lack of a waist and about how her stomach stood out farther than her chest when she gained too much weight. When family members asked about her health, she always replied that the doctor said she was fine. Her blood sugar was a little high, but it wasn't diabetes. Her cholesterol was a little high, but not in the danger zone. Her blood pressure was also just a little high, which she was treating by taking a diuretic, a 'water pill'. Earlier that night she died, she had said she felt 'not right'. She hadn't been able to sleep, and paced around the house. She hadn't recognised the early symptoms of heart attack.

If this book had been written just six months earlier, Ginny might still be alive. Although she had no single, glaring risk factor, all the little signs added up to a heart attack waiting to happen. She didn't recognise it, and unfortunately, neither did her doctor. There are medications that could have saved her life. Or perhaps she could have had surgery to unblock her arteries. Maybe if she knew how much her apple shape and smoking were affecting her health, she would have changed her lifestyle, adjusted her diet, stopped smoking. Maybe if she had known that most women who have heart attacks don't experience the same symptoms as men, she might have called for help sooner. Maybe . . . if.

Heart disease is the number-one killer of women. It strikes down more of us than all cancers put together, including lung cancer and breast cancer. Yet most women are oddly unconcerned about heart disease and its fatal or debilitating sister, stroke. Maybe that's because we psychologically associate 'heart attack' with men, and therefore we feel immune. Or maybe it's because the public health emphasis has been put on educating women about the value of mammograms for early detection of breast cancer. That campaign sought to spur us into action by instilling fear, and it worked. Women tend to wildly overestimate their risk of developing breast cancer, but they barely give a thought to heart disease. It's wonderful that women are finally marking breast cancer screening dates on their calendars. But I'd like to see the same level of awareness applied to cardiovascular disease. No fear, just the facts. No more 'maybe if'.

Most women are oddly unconcerned about heart disease and stroke – perhaps because we associate 'heart attack' with men. But make no mistake about it. Heart disease is the number-one killer of women.

Like Type 2 diabetes, cardiovascular disease is highly preventable and controllable. It's just a matter of understanding what happens in the body to start the cascade of problems that can eventually result in heart attack, and then breaking in to stop or reverse the process. Think of it like riding down a steep hill on a bicycle. There are many different ways you can stop the slide, even if the decline is brisk – you're not doomed to crash at the bottom. And if you work hard enough, you can even turn that bicycle around and head back up to the crest. Of course it's better not to go down that road in the first place!

CARDIOVASCULAR DISEASE

Cardiovascular disease is a term that encompasses a variety of disorders that have to do with the heart (*cardio*) and with blood vessels (*vasculo*) throughout the body. The most common disorders are caused when a blockage occurs in an artery, cutting off the blood supply to a portion of the body.

Blood flow becomes blocked if there is a buildup of *plaque* along the inside walls of the arteries, a process known as *atherosclerosis*. Plaque is a hardened mixture of oxidised cholesterol and other fatty substances, cellular waste and calcium. If enough plaque builds up, the artery walls can narrow to the point where blood flow is weak, hindered or entirely blocked. This is equivalent to the atherosclerotic/ rusted pipes in my old house. The water in the shower barely dribbles out, and it doesn't take much to stop it altogether – just a little change in water pressure, such as if the dishwasher is running. And the body works similarly. If we have blocked arteries so that the blood just dribbles through, a little diversion of blood – such as to muscles during exercise – can stop the flow to the heart entirely. That's why many heart attacks occur during or after vigorous exercise or other exertion. Sometimes, pieces of the plaque break off and travel in the bloodstream. If those hunks of waxlike substance are large enough, they can dam an artery and block blood flow. More often, the plaque becomes unstable and ruptures, and a blood clot forms at the rupture site. The result is the same – blocked blood flow. Without blood, body parts become damaged, fail and eventually die.

The specific damage caused by the blockage depends on what part of the body is affected. If blood flow to the heart is blocked, the result is a heart attack, also called *myocardial infarction.* If blood flow to the brain is blocked, the result is a stroke, also called *cerebrovascular accident* or *brain attack.* If blood flow to more distant body parts, such as the feet, is blocked, the result is *peripheral vascular disease,* which may require amputation to remove the 'dead' body part.

So the important questions for preventing cardiovascular disease are: (1) Why does plaque develop? and (2) How do we stop it?

Plaque and Heart Disease

Plaque is believed to start when the inside walls of the arteries are damaged. We're used to thinking of our bodies as relatively tough – skin and bones are durable and made to take the punishment of living. The linings of our blood vessels are much more delicate, thin silk instead of denim. The main causes of damage are high blood pressure, high blood glucose (which happens with the metabolic syndrome and diabetes), high levels of triglycerides or low-density lipoprotein (LDL) cholesterol, and tobacco smoke.

Once the damage occurs, the body tries to heal itself by activating inflammatory processes, the same processes that cause healing after you cut your skin. The body reacts by releasing inflammation-related body chemicals called *cytokines,* such as *tumour necrosis factor-alpha* (TNF-α). These cytokines play a role in immunity, so they are not bad in general. For example, TNF-α is one of the body's natural cancer fighters, as its name suggests – 'necrosis' means death. But if levels of these cytokines remain elevated, the long-term effects can be harmful. For example, TNF-α alters the ability of insulin receptors to accept insulin, leading to glucose intolerance and insulin insensitivity, which leads to high blood glucose, which leads to damage to the blood vessel walls, which results in atherosclerosis and heart disease. TNF-α also helps to make the cell walls 'stickier', which starts the process of plaque build-up. Of course, the damage to the cell walls and plaque itself trigger even more inflammatory chemicals to be made and released. It becomes a downhill ride as inflammatory factors build upon each other to create a hostile environment in our bodies. The final insult is that inflammation not only starts the process of atherosclerosis, it also makes the plaque more fragile, and therefore more likely to break off and cause a blockage downstream, or to rupture and cause a blood clot.

C-reactive Protein and Inflammation

The body also produces a mysterious substance called *C-reactive protein* (CRP). No one knows exactly what CRP does in the body, but whenever there is inflammation, the amount of CRP goes up. Because of this relationship, we use CRP as a *marker* for inflammation. Because inflammation itself can't be directly measured, CRP is used as a shortcut to help us determine whether inflammation is present. If CRP is elevated and there is no other obvious cause of inflammation, such as an infection or autoimmune disease, then atherosclerosis is probably there, too.

Studies have shown that CRP levels predict heart attack risk better than cholesterol levels, with higher levels of CRP resulting in a higher risk of cardiovascular disease. Measuring cholesterol misses about half of all cases of potential heart attack, but CRP catches them all. (While all heart attack patients have an elevated CRP level, elevated CRP doesn't necessarily mean heart attack – it could mean any inflammation-related disorders, including rheumatoid arthritis, lupus, recent surgery or an active infection.)

A woman with the metabolic syndrome is twice as likely to have a heart attack as healthy women; but a woman with the metabolic syndrome *and* high levels of CRP is *four times more likely to suffer a heart attack.* Among women aged 65 or older, the risk of cardiovascular disease was eight times higher in women with a high level of CRP (>3.0 mg/L) versus a low level of CRP (<1.0 mg/L). So by measuring CRP, we can catch those high-risk individuals who otherwise might have fallen through the health care cracks. They can take steps to prevent further damage and very possibly save their lives.

The answer to the question of how we stop the process of atherosclerosis is a little more complex. The quick answer is easy – fix all the stuff that leads to inflammation. Stop smoking. Keep blood pressure low. Keep triglycerides and LDL cholesterol low. Control blood glucose levels. Treat chronic infections, such as periodontitis. Basically, do everything you can to prevent additional inflammation in the body. That includes paying attention to body shape.

BODY SHAPE AND CARDIOVASCULAR DISEASE

Physicians have come to view obesity as the greatest threat to heart health. But as you probably know by now, it is not overall body fat, but the distribution of the fat that matters. Again, recent research has shown that most of the blame should fall on visceral fat.

Fat of all kinds contributes to inflammation by secreting pro-inflammatory hormones and cytokines, including TNF-α. (Cytokines that are produced by fat tissue are called *adipokines*.) But visceral fat is much more metabolically active than pear-zone subcutaneous fat, and it releases these adipokines in greater concentrations. Plus, researchers have discovered that visceral fat and CRP go hand in hand. The larger the waist, the higher the levels of CRP, regardless of overall body weight. This means that apple-shaped women generally have more ongoing, low-level inflammation than pear-shaped women – raising their risk of heart disease even in the absence of any other risk factor.

Aside from affecting inflammation, visceral fat also increases triglycerides and LDL levels, and decreases HDL levels. As discussed in chapter 5, visceral fat also increases the risk of the metabolic syndrome and diabetes, which directly cause damage to the blood vessels, starting the downhill roll towards heart disease. The greater the stores of visceral fat, the worse all the risks are.

This equates to all apple-shaped women – whether they are lean or overweight – having an increased risk for all cardiovascular diseases. Studies have shown that having an apple shape increases the risk for stroke threefold, regardless of body weight. Apple-shaped women also face an increased risk for heart attack. The Nurses' Health Study, which tracked more than 44,000 women for eight years, showed that women with a waist-to-hip ratio (WHR) of 0.88 or higher were three times more likely to have a heart attack than women with a WHR of less than 0.72, *regardless of total body weight*. And the higher the WHR, or the higher the waist circumference, the greater the risk.

Researchers in Australia compared body mass index (BMI) to waist circumference and WHR to see which measure was best able to predict death from cardiovascular disease. They followed more than 9,200 adults, ages 20 to 69, for 11 years. In that time, there were 473 deaths. After analysing all the health information, they discovered that WHR was the best predictor of death from heart attack or stroke. Beginning with a WHR of 0.80 – the criterion for being labelled an apple-shaped woman – the risk increased dramatically. And again, the higher the WHR, the higher the risk. In fact, *the risk associated with having an apple shape was higher than the individual risks for high cholesterol, high blood pressure or smoking*.

Irregular periods are another warning sign. Research has shown that women with a history of having had irregular periods between ages 20 and 35 have about a 50 per cent greater risk of heart attack overall compared with women who had regular periods. And the more irregular the periods, the greater the risk of heart disease, regardless of weight. Why? No one really knows, but it is probably a marker for hormonal imbalance in general, and it most likely has to do with the predominance of androgen. Women with PCOS have an androgen predominance, and they also have irregular periods. Apple-shaped women typically have irregular periods, and their visceral fat gives them a slightly higher androgen level. We also know that apple-shaped women and women with PCOS have a greater risk of heart disease. There's a good chance that the hormones related to body shape are also connected with heart disease. Although there is nothing you can do to change your menstrual history, this information can be a valuable personal tool, an added push to visit the doctor if you had irregular menstruation.

Pear-shaped women will be happy to note that thigh fat is related to higher levels of HDL cholesterol, which we know is associated with a lower risk of heart disease. Studies have also shown that thigh fat is associated with lower levels of triglycerides and LDL cholesterol, and lower blood pressure. This means that 'thunder thighs' actually may protect pear-shaped women from the risk factors of cardiovascular disease!

HEART ATTACKS: THE RED FLAGS

Heart attacks occur most often in older women, but that doesn't mean younger women can ignore the warning signs. One woman that stands out in my memory is Joanne, a woman who died of heart disease at age 44. Joanne was not a patient of mine, but I had an opportunity to review her case after she died. Joanne saw her primary care physician regularly, and got occasional blood tests as part of her annual physical examination. Like Ginny, Joanne was always told that everything was 'fine'. When I looked over her records, I saw that her blood glucose levels were often higher than 120, her blood pressure was high, and her triglycerides were in the 250 range. But because she was relatively young, and because her total cholesterol was in the 'safe' range of about 200, and because doctors don't worry as much about triglycerides, her physician wasn't concerned. Joanne thought she was healthy.

What should have been obvious to her physician was that Joanne was overweight and apple-shaped. I never met her, but even I could see her large 'triglyceride waist' in photographs that her family showed me. She also had a lot of stress – two jobs to support three teenagers and an ailing husband who was on disability. She made a doctor's appointment when she noticed a 'heaviness' in her chest and mentioned that she had general discomfort and shortness of breath that came on at odd times – not always when she exerted herself. Her doctor called it 'atypical chest pain' and blamed it on stress from overwork. She was advised to relieve some stress by walking, which is usually a good recommendation. However, Joanne started walking with her daughter in her very hilly neighbourhood, pressing onward despite more and more chest discomfort. Everyone assumed it was because she was out of shape.

Joanne had a heart attack and died eight months later after many attempts to clear her blocked arteries. Even when her death was near, Joanne's doctors didn't seem to understand exactly how sick she was. When I had a chance to review her records, it turned out that she had had diabetes for years (her doctor never brought her abnormal fasting glucose of 130 to 150 to her attention), and her blood glucose went out of control after the heart attack. Because of the diabetes, her arteries were seriously blocked, and the angioplasty didn't 'take' – the arteries became reblocked very quickly. At that point, she should have had bypass surgery, but her cardiologist encouraged her to keep trying the noninvasive, but ultimately unsuccessful methods. She should have sought a second opinion, but she trusted her doctor to make the best decisions for her.

If Joanne had been a man, chances are her symptoms would have been taken much more seriously. Her feeling of chest heaviness would probably have been correctly diagnosed as acute coronary insufficiency, also called unstable angina, and she would have been started on treatment to prevent a heart attack, including a daily aspirin, a beta-blocker and long-acting nitroglycerin. In addition, her diabetes might have been detected and given the attention it deserved, and she would have been given a statin drug to control her cholesterol. Joanne was given nothing but a refill of her prescription tranquiliser to treat her so-called stress disease.

In general, women are incredibly underdiagnosed and undertreated for heart disease. Part of it is our own fault – we don't want to 'bother' the doctor with our symptoms, or we're too busy to make an appointment, or we believe that heart attacks are strictly a man's problem. But part of it is the fault of the medical community, which is still unfamiliar with the language of body shape. Doctors have not yet begun to check for the 'triglyceride waist', nor do they recognise the different health risks for apple- and pear-shaped women. Sadly, many doctors are still more willing to write women a prescription for Valium or an antidepressant than to give them a stress test to check for cardiovascular disease.

This means that we have to be more willing to visit the doctor when we aren't feeling well, and we have to understand the symptoms of heart disease that women experience. Don't wait for 'classic symptoms' of angina or heart disease. Many women – and men, for that matter – don't experience the textbook signs, such as chest tightness that comes on slowly with exertion, pain that may radiate down the left arm or into the jaw. Women often feel something much more vague: an awareness of heavier breathing or shortness of breath with exertion, or a feeling of nausea or generalised fatigue, or a heaviness in the chest. But one thing is certain, women know the messages from their bodies. We know when we feel well, and we know when something does not feel quite right. We may not know the causes, but we know when our bodies are talking to us. One of our biggest goals is to learn to listen!

CONTROLLING INFLAMMATION AND CARDIOVASCULAR DISEASE

Although all women, apple-shaped and pear-shaped, can develop cardiovascular disease, pear-shaped women are more likely to have isolated risk factors, such as high cholesterol or high blood pressure. Apple-shaped women are more likely to have the ominous *combination* of multiple risk factors. Combining risk factors has a synergistic effect, so that the risks don't merely add to each other, they multiply. And the effect of each risk factor is worse for apple-shaped women than for pear-shaped women. As a result, an apple-shaped woman needs to eliminate or reduce each risk factor in order to preserve her health. Start small, but work diligently. Everything you do to lower any of the proinflammatory factors in your life will help reduce your risk of cardiovascular disease.

Smoking

The number one recommendation on every physician's hit list for heart disease is to stop smoking. Within months after you stop smoking, your risk of heart disease begins to drop. After three to five years, your risk will be the same as that of a nonsmoker. Talk with your doctor about some of the new aids available for stopping smoking.

Diet and Exercise

Follow the diet and exercise programmes for apple-shaped women in Part 3. The recommendations are designed to be heart-healthy. By losing fat and girth from around your waist, you'll reduce the concentrations of proinflammatory adipokines, reduce triglycerides and

LDL cholesterol, and raise HDL cholesterol – all of which will lower your overall risk of cardiovascular disease.

Medications

Use medications if necessary. As much as we want to do things 'naturally', prescription drugs can be lifesavers. Remember, there are many different medications that can treat your cardiac risk factors or heart disease. If you have problems with one medication, talk with your doctor to find out which alternatives might be right for you. Don't stop taking your medication without discussing it with your doctor, and don't give up on perfect control. There are always new options to help you be as heart-healthy as possible.

Medications for Apple-Shaped Women

◆ **High blood pressure.** Don't believe the 'old wives' tale' my grandmother used to tell me, that a normal blood pressure should be '100 plus your age'. In general, the lower your blood pressure, the better. Normal blood pressure is defined as *less than* 120/80. High blood pressure, or hypertension, is blood pressure that is 140/90 or higher. All numbers in between are classified as prehypertension and should be taken as a warning sign that heart disease has begun. Apple-shaped women who have diabetes should set their blood pressure goal to be under 130/80. If you have diabetes with kidney disease or protein in your urine, your blood pressure needs to be even lower – 125/80.

For apple-shaped women, the best blood pressure medications have been ACE (angiotensin-converting enzyme) inhibitors, such as Carace or Zestril (lisinopril), Innovace (enalapril), or Tritace (ramipril). Research has shown that ACE inhibitors can reduce the risks of both cardiovascular disease and renal disease, which can be especially important for women with the metabolic syndrome or diabetes. I believe that almost every apple-shaped woman with high blood pressure and diabetes should take an ACE inhibitor. The newest blood pressure medications are the angiotensin receptor blockers (ARBs), such as Cozaar (losartan). ARBs seem to be just as effective as ACE inhibitors, but they cause fewer allergic reactions and may work better at warding off diabetes-related kidney disease. Although ACE inhibitors are still the first-line therapy for hypertension, more and more research suggests that ARBs may soon become the medication of choice.

Many doctors like to start patients on diuretics before starting ACE inhibitors, but I think it should be the other way around – diuretics should be taken by apple-shaped women only if blood pressure cannot be controlled with ACE inhibitors. That's because the most commonly prescribed diuretics, the 'thiazides' (including Dyazide and Moduretic), can cause an elevation of blood glucose. Women who have the metabolic syndrome or diet-controlled diabetes may find themselves needing to begin taking an oral diabetes medication once they start taking these medications. If you must take a thiazide diuretic to control blood pressure, you should have regular blood glucose checks to monitor your levels.

Another good blood pressure medication that I sometimes recommend for apple-shaped women who also have angina or a history of heart attack is a beta-blocker, which controls blood pressure and regulates heart rhythm. Research has shown that beta-blockers – such as Inderal (propranolol), Tenormin (atenolol) and Lopresor (metoprolol) – can prevent sudden death in a patient with heart disease. However, beta-blockers – like diuretics – can lead to insulin resistance and worsen blood glucose levels. ACE inhibitors and ARBs are my first choices for controlling blood pressure in apple-shaped women.

◆ **High blood fats.** Apple-shaped women need to shoot for a target goal of LDL cholesterol under 100, especially if they have other cardiovascular risk factors, such as diabetes, or the metabolic syndrome. The first-line treatment choice should be a statin medication – always in addition to, not instead of, the diet and exercise programme in Part 3. Along with lowering cholesterol, statins also work to reduce inflammation. Statin medications include Zocor (simvastatin), Lipitor (atorvastatin) and Lipostat (pravastatin). These medications are still terribly underused; a lot of heart attacks could be prevented if doctors would prescribe statins to at-risk apple-shaped women with high LDL cholesterol. New guidelines suggest shooting for a target goal of LDL cholesterol under 70 for people who have an extremely increased risk, such as having had a previous heart attack.

For apple-shaped women who also have high triglycerides (over 150 mg/dL) and low HDL cholesterol (under 50 mg/dL), I recommend taking 1,000 milligrams of fish oil daily. Fish oil has been shown to decrease triglycerides and lower CRP in women who take it daily, and it may also help raise HDL cholesterol and reduce the risk of fatal heart arrhythmias. Fish oil capsules are available wherever vitamin supplements are sold. All brands seem to be similar, so choose based on price or personal preference. I'll warn you that some people find that their skin or breath starts to smell a little fishy after taking the supplements. Still, it's worth a try.

I also prescribe niacin or Lopid (gemfibrozil) to control high triglycerides, but cautiously in women who are already taking statins. The combination of medications can lead to more and rather serious side effects of muscle breakdown and pain. If you must take that combination, you'll need close and careful monitoring, although I have only seen serious muscle problems from statins in women with the metabolic syndrome.

◆ **Cardiovascular protection.** Apple-shaped women should consider taking an aspirin a day for general cardiovascular protection, especially if they have the metabolic syndrome or diabetes. The small dose of a single 'baby aspirin', just 81 milligrams per day, helps thin the blood so that clots are less likely to form, and it also acts as an anti-inflammatory. (Of course, you don't have to buy special 81 milligram tablets if the larger sizes are less expensive – just cut the larger 325 milligram tablets into four doses.) Do not take aspirin if you have any trouble with blood clotting, or if you are taking warfarin or other blood-thinning medication – too much blood-thinning medication may also be dangerous if you have some injury that needs clotting to stop the bleeding. You should also avoid aspirin if you have had allergic reactions to aspirin in the past, or if you have asthma or nasal polyps, which sometimes indicate a possible aspirin allergy. Always, always, *always* talk with your doctor before starting to take aspirin or other over-the-counter medication for disease prevention.

Medications for Pear-Shaped Women

After menopause, pear-shaped women can turn into apple-shaped women. With this shape shift, they assume all the same risks that go along with having too much visceral fat and may find that they require the same medications as apple-shaped women. Although pear-shaped women have a much lower risk of heart disease than apple-shaped women, they may still need to consider treatment for hypertension, high cholesterol, and general cardiovascular protection.

◆ **High blood pressure.** Pear-shaped women with high blood pressure can safely begin taking one of the hydrochlorothiazide or other 'thiazide' diuretics (such as Dyazide or Moduretic) as their first choice for high blood pressure. These medications have the added benefits of reducing fluid retention, which may help prevent varicose veins, and improving bone mass density, thereby reducing the risk of fractures from osteoporosis – both important concerns for pear-shaped women.

◆ **High blood fats.** Pear-shaped women are less likely to have high triglycerides or low HDL cholesterol. However, they may experience high LDL cholesterol as they go through menopause. The target goal for LDL cholesterol for healthy pear-shaped women is under 130. They can usually achieve this goal through changes in diet and exercise without a need for medication.

◆ **Cardiovascular protection.** Unless a pear-shaped woman has other risk factors for heart disease, such as the metabolic syndrome or type 2 diabetes, she is less likely to benefit from treatment with aspirin. However, beginning low-dose hormone therapy (HT) at menopause may help protect pear-shaped women from developing heart disease (see details in chapter 4). Thousands of women and years of observational studies have shown that healthy women, most likely pear-shaped, were able to reduce their risks for heart attack and death by half by starting to take low-dose HT early in menopause. They also usually have an improvement in blood fats. Talk with your doctor about the risks and benefits if you think you might like to try HT.

HEALTH SOLUTIONS ARE EASIER THAN YOU THINK

I'm hoping that you are beginning to see that we're talking about a huge, multilayered, interconnected group of physiological effects that all stem from visceral fat. Many apple-shaped women I talk to feel overwhelmed by all their additional disease risk. Please keep in mind that most of these additional risks will disappear if you reduce your stores of visceral fat by reducing your waist. It's like pulling that single thread that ends up unravelling an entire sweater — it shouldn't be that simple, but it is. Sure, there will always be genetic factors that contribute to disease risk, but you can't control them. You can control visceral fat! If you learn nothing more from this book, I hope you remember that a few centimetres around your waist may mean the difference between early death and good health.

Action Items for Chapter 6:
Heart Disease, Stroke and Inflammation

◆ Don't be a heart attack waiting to happen.

1. Schedule an appointment with your physician to discuss your risk factors and concerns and get any additional testing you may need. At a minimum, you'll want to have your fasting glucose and fasting lipids tested. Record all test results on your Body Shape Health Log (page 328).

2. Ask about having your blood levels of CRP checked. I recommend this to all women with diabetes or the metabolic syndrome, all apple-shaped women over age 40, and pear-shaped women with a waist circumference larger than 90cm (35½in). It is also a good idea to have a baseline CRP measurement before starting hormone therapy (HT) after menopause. Some oral HT medications raise CRP, so you'll want to monitor what happens.

3. Set treatment goals with your physician for each risk factor – blood glucose, LDL cholesterol, HDL cholesterol, triglycerides and CRP.

4. Discuss what lifestyle changes you have begun (including the programmes in this book), and discuss which medications might help you achieve your goals quicker and more easily.

5. Discuss how frequently you should be monitored and what monitoring you can do on your own. For example, many women buy a simple blood pressure monitor they can use at home.

◆ If you are an apple-shaped woman and have high blood glucose, high triglycerides, low HDL cholesterol or high LDL cholesterol, don't 'wait and see'. Take action by asking your doctor for an aggressive course of treatment. And don't be afraid to take medications to get your numbers in line. You can always stop taking medications once you lose a few centimetres from your waist or start exercising to control these risk factors.

◆ Keep a journal of all heart-related symptoms, including unusual fatigue, chest pain, chest tightness or heaviness, or shortness of breath that occurs with exertion or stress or after a heavy meal. Your doctor will want to know all the details so that he or she can make a precise diagnosis, recommend the right diagnostic tests and prescribe the best treatment.

◆ Ask for a cardiac stress test *if*: (1) you are having symptoms of heart disease; (2) you are an apple-shaped women with two or more of the following risk factors for heart disease: the metabolic syndrome, type 2 diabetes, high LDL cholesterol, high triglycerides, low HDL cholesterol; (3) you are a sedentary woman over age 40 getting ready to start an exercise programme. The cardiac stress test is an electrocardiogram that is taken while you are exercising on a treadmill. The purpose is to find out how your heart performs while you're exerting yourself and to learn if you could already have blocked heart arteries.

◆ Find a 'health partner', someone you trust who will listen to your health concerns, go to doctor appointments with you if necessary, and generally be your touchstone. Sometimes just talking about your concerns with a friend can help you recognise the seriousness of your symptoms. An outside perspective may help you decide to see the doctor sooner rather than later.

◆ Nurture a sense of calm. Regardless of whatever other risk factors you have, being angry, hostile, impatient or in a perpetual state of time urgency (always fighting the clock) increases the risk of heart attack. Add impatience to other risk factors, and your life just became riskier.

Take to Heart ...

◆ Regardless of whatever else you do in life, you are the number-one expert in at least one area: how you feel. By the time you live 20, 30, 40, 50 or more years in the same body, you know when something isn't right. You know when the daily fatigue is beyond what you typically expect. You know when there's an unfamiliar pain or ache you can't explain. You know when your health is no longer status quo. When that happens, see your doctor. There are many possible reasons for a change in health, and you want the chance to treat any significant disease early. If your doctor blames it on stress or indigestion or depression or your weight or any other tangential factor in your life without running any tests, try to change to another doctor. If the problem persists after you try a treatment, go back to the doctor and let her know that you are still concerned. You are the expert. Don't stop searching for answers until you feel better.

◆ Part of being a woman seems to be having an unending amount of energy and caring for other people. Try to tap into some of that wellspring for yourself. I've seen patients who wait far too long to come in for an appointment because they are too busy. Along with either working full-time or caring for children, they have to attend PTA meetings, work overtime, do a school run, take a night class, run errands, cook meals and perform all the other myriad chores that seem to fall specifically to women. The problem is that your carefully planned schedule of events falls apart if you become seriously ill. Your personal health care deserves at least as much time as your personal hair care. Strive to take care of yourself at least as well as you take care of your friends and family.

CHAPTER 7

Breast and Endometrial Cancer

Cancer is a dark mystery. It is a nightmare that seems to bubble up from nowhere. Those who are affected feel invaded, which is why many people are surprised to learn that cancer starts from normal body cells. Something mutates them, alters them, sets them off, causing them to no longer act like normal body cells. At any given moment, we all have thousands of mutated precancerous cells in our bodies, but only rarely do any of them become truly cancerous. Most of the time, our immune system takes care of those rebel cells, clearing them out like so much rubbish. But if the cancerous cells start to multiply, they can overwhelm the body's defences and we become sick.

The keys to solving the cancer mystery lie in discovering what makes a cell mutate in the first place, and then what allows it to multiply and grow. If we knew that, then virtually every case of cancer could be prevented or stopped before it caused serious damage. We know some pieces of the puzzle. We know, for example, that radiation from sunlight can cause cells to mutate – and the result can be skin cancer. We know that toxins from cigarette smoke can cause lung cells to mutate – and the result can be lung cancer. We know that infection with *Helicobacter pylori* bacteria can cause mutations in the lining of stomach cells – and the result can be stomach cancer. We know that a persistent infection with some strains of the human papillomavirus (HPV) is the sole cause of cervical cancer. Even for these factors we know about, the result is not always the same. Not everyone who smokes will develop lung cancer. Not everyone who basks in the sun will develop skin cancer. Most people with HPV infection won't get cervical cancer. The potential is there, but other factors tip the balance for each individual – cancer, or no cancer. But most of the time, we have no idea what causes cells to mutate in a particular individual, or whether those mutated cells will grow into cancer. That frightening unpredictability is what makes cancer the great bogeyman of health care.

Even though exact cancer predictions aren't possible, scientists can make some educated guesses based on research. In order to appreciate these findings, it's helpful to understand how the research is conducted. Some of the information is based on studies of what happens when animals are exposed to potentially cancer-causing agents. That gives us background information about how it might work in people, but it can't tell us everything. People and animals are similar, but not the same. Right now, scientists have the ability to cure mice of just about every kind of cancer imaginable. But when those same cures are applied to people, they don't work. To understand what might cause cancer in people, we have to gather clues from those who already have the disease – how are they different from people who don't have cancer? With the help of statistics, researchers try to find behavioural, genetic or environmental factors that are more common among people with a specific type of cancer than among healthy people. For example, hundreds of studies have shown that the main difference between women with lung cancer and women without lung cancer is cigarette smoking. It is said, then, that lung cancer *is related to* smoking. We can't prove that smoking *caused* the lung cancer, but we know that there is a strong association.

There are no absolutes when it comes to cancer.

I feel it's important to explain this because cancer really is still a mystery. In identical twins who have the exact same genetic susceptibility to breast cancer, it is possible that only one of the twins will go on to develop the disease. Chances are we'll never know exactly why. The best we can do is understand what factors are somehow related to cancer and then do all we can to do the opposite. Of course, that's easier said than done. Knowing what to do is always much easier than actually doing it. Researchers estimate that one-third of all cancers could be prevented if no one smoked. That's a whole lot of cancer – and yet people still smoke. You've got to do what you can, but even if you do everything right, you may still get cancer. And if you do everything wrong, some of you will avoid cancer. There are no absolutes when it comes to cancer. In this chapter, I will let you know what the current research says about body shape and cancer and what actions I recommend to stack the odds in your favour.

BREAST CANCER

The cancer women fear most is breast cancer. Lung cancer claims more lives, but breast cancer is the disease that makes us wake up in a cold sweat. It is a relatively common cancer among women, striking about 32,000 women and killing about 12,000 women in Britain each year. Most women are so worried about the threat of breast cancer that they would do anything to prevent it. Some women who learn that they have genetic mutations that make breast cancer all but certain opt to have both their breasts removed, a procedure known as prophylactic double mastectomy. For the average woman, however, medical science has very little to offer in terms of prevention.

Breast Cancer: The Risk Factors

We know some of the factors that are related to breast cancer, and most of them are not under our control. Some of the risk is genetic, so if any blood member in your family – from either your mother's or your father's side – has had breast cancer, you should automatically consider yourself at increased risk. If your mother or a sister has had breast cancer, you have an even higher risk. And if multiple close family members have had breast cancer, your risk may be four or five times higher than that of the average woman. We also know that the risk for breast cancer increases as we get older. Having children seems to lower the risk of developing breast cancer, and the more children you have, the lower your risk. Tall women have a higher risk of breast cancer than short women. And the younger you are when you get your first period, or the older you are when you reach menopause, the higher your overall risk of breast cancer.

Beyond that, the causes of breast cancer are sketchy. As discussed in chapter 4, taking hormone therapy for menopausal symptoms for more than five years has been shown to increase the risk of breast cancer by about 26 per cent. And some research has linked alcohol to an increased risk for breast cancer.

Interestingly, the common thread running through all these seemingly disparate factors is oestrogen. Alcohol increases the amount of oestrogen in the blood, hormone therapy is all about oestrogen, pregnancy lowers oestrogen levels in the body and the longer in life you menstruate, the more oestrogen you'll have cycling in your body. Of course, another source of oestrogen in women's bodies is fat.

Breast Cancer and Obesity

Obesity has consistently been shown to be related to an increased risk of breast cancer in postmenopausal women, but not in premenopausal women. Premenopausal women who are overweight don't seem to have any increased risk of breast cancer. The problem comes from weight gain throughout adulthood. Can you remember what you weighed when you were 18 years old? Studies show that the more weight you gain after age 18, the higher your risk for breast cancer – women who gain 20kg (3 stone, 3lb) double their risk. This is thought to be related to the amount of oestrogen produced in fat tissue, and overweight women can have double the amount of oestrogen as lean women. And because women tend to put on most of their weight during pregnancies and after menopause, those kilos will probably be visceral fat, which goes to form an apple shape. We know that visceral fat creates the more powerful form of oestrogen, so it would be logical to assume that apple-shaped women have a greater risk of developing breast cancer than pear-shaped women.

Breast Cancer and Body Shape

Indeed, logic prevails. Some researchers have looked specifically at the relationship of body shape to breast cancer risk. Individually, the studies have been confusing and sometimes conflicting. One study looked at nearly 2,500 women, half with breast cancer, half without cancer. Researchers discovered that body shape had no relationship to breast cancer among premenopausal women. But among post-menopausal women, those who had the highest waist-to-hip ratio (WHR) had a 40 per cent greater risk of breast cancer than women with the lowest WHR, regardless of how much physical activity the women engaged in over their lives and regardless of diet. In the Nurses' Health Study, there was no relationship between body shape and breast cancer in premenopausal women. However, postmenopausal women with the highest WHR and the highest waist circumference had about a 35 per cent increased risk of breast cancer, compared with women who had the lowest WHR and waist circumference.

On the other hand, a few researchers have claimed to find that even premenopausal apple-shaped women have a higher risk. In 2002, researchers from Toronto, Canada, did a meta-analysis of all the published literature on the relationship between weight and breast cancer. This type of analysis pools all the data from the various individual studies, gives standard definitions to the variables, and then looks at the results. These researchers found that apple-shaped women have about a 60 per cent increased risk of breast cancer overall compared with pear-shaped women. In their analysis, the risk was slightly greater for premenopausal women.

Because we don't know exactly how the women in these studies were chosen, when their weight was gained and lots of other contributing variables, it is difficult to understand exactly what is happening in premenopausal women. It may be that other factors that cause such a devastating disease in young women overwhelm the weight issue. What seems clear, however, is that weight – particularly in the apple zone – is a major contributor to breast cancer risk in postmenopausal women.

You can reduce your risk of breast cancer
kilo by kilo, centimetre by centimetre.

The good news is that the increased risk due to weight may be entirely reversible. One fascinating study followed more than 21,000 women for seven years. Based on the expected number of breast cancers in a group this large, the researchers were able to determine the effects of *losing weight* on breast cancer risk. Women who intentionally lost 9kg (10lb) or more reduced their risk for breast cancer by nearly 20 per cent – about 2 per cent per kilo. And if those women reached their target weight so that they were no longer overweight, their risk was identical to lean women who never were overweight. This is encouraging and very optimistic news for every woman. We've never before been offered any concrete way to reduce the risk of this dreaded disease, and here it is: you can reduce your risk of breast cancer kilo by kilo, centimetre by centimetre.

ENDOMETRIAL CANCER

Endometrial cancer, which affects the inside lining of the uterus, strikes only about 2 per cent of U.S. women, and yet it is the most common reproductive cancer. It is highly preventable, and because it can cause irregular bleeding – even in women after menopause – it is usually detected early enough to allow for a complete cure.

During a normal menstrual cycle, the high levels of oestrogen allow the endometrium to grow and thicken in preparation for pregnancy. If a fertilised egg does not become implanted, rising progesterone causes the thickened lining to be shed, which culminates in menstrual bleeding. In a woman with endometrial cancer, the lining doesn't shed, usually because there is no balance of progesterone to mature the lining cells or signal the time to shed the lining. Instead, the lining continues to grow and thicken, resulting in cancer.

So again, the hormonal balance is critically important. If a woman wants to take hormone therapy after menopause, oestrogen is given to ease her menopausal symptoms, but progesterone is given periodically to mature the lining and to cause any endometrial lining to be shed. Women who no longer have a uterus can take oestrogen alone, because they obviously have no risk of endometrial cancer.

Endometrial Cancer: The Risk Factors

As with breast cancer, there are many uncontrollable factors related to endometrial cancer. The risk is lower for women with more children, women who begin menstruating later, and women who go through menopause earlier. The risk is higher for women with diabetes and for women who have irregular menstrual periods. Although early research found that the risk was higher for overweight women, later research has almost uniformly found that, once again, visceral fat is to blame for the increased risk. Apple-shaped women have double the risk of endometrial cancer compared with pear-shaped women, regardless of their overall weight. When you consider that apple-shaped women are more likely to have irregular periods, this, too, makes sense.

The same study that examined the effects of weight loss on breast cancer risk found that losing 9kg (10lb) reduced the risk of endometrial cancer by 4 per cent. But when you consider that diabetes is also a risk factor for endometrial cancer, and that weight loss can prevent diabetes, the overall benefit of weight loss may be even larger than this study suggests.

Stories of Endometrial Cancer

Although endometrial cancer is usually caught early, sometimes a woman has to fight for a proper diagnosis. A prime example is Fran Drescher, the actress who starred in the television show *The Nanny*. I had a chance to speak with her at a Women in Government conference – she was a patient advocate and I was the physician on a panel about women's gynaecologic cancers and importance of early diagnosis and treatment. She was thin and gorgeous, but because she was in a trouser suit, I couldn't tell if she was apple- or pear-shaped and didn't get a chance to ask her. (Believe me, I am not shy about asking women where they carry their weight!) Her endometrial cancer had been diagnosed when she was in her mid-40s, after being missed for two years and by seven doctors. After her television series folded, she began complaining of midcycle bleeding and spotting. Plus, she just didn't feel right. She got really worried when she began to experience pain with intercourse. She visited a total of seven doctors, all of whom missed the diagnosis. She even had an ultrasound done in a doctor's office, but perhaps the wrong technique was used, or the technician wasn't properly skilled. It didn't pick up the cancer.

Ms. Drescher's message, which I share, is that if you have midcycle spotting, insist on *vaginal probe ultrasound* and an *endometrial biopsy.* (You may need to have this done privately.) A typical ultrasound is done with a device that looks a bit like a cell phone that passes over your belly. A vaginal probe is a painless procedure that is done with a wand that is partly inserted into the vagina. An endometrial biopsy requires the doctor to enter your cervix and take a sample scraping from the lining of your uterus. In Ms. Drescher's case, no one did the simple endometrial biopsy until the eighth doctor, and even then only at the insistence of her sister, a nurse.

Why did so many doctors miss her cancer? Ms. Drescher says it was because everyone assumed that she was under a lot of stress – the television series was cancelled, plus she left her long-time husband and was living alone – so the doctors simply thought she was perimeno-pausal (even though perimenopause shouldn't cause midcycle spotting or spotting after sex). By the time the cancer was finally diagnosed, it was more advanced. The good news is that after a radical hysterectomy, she has been cancer free since 2001, and she feels great. My message to you is that if a famous actress seeing seven doctors can have endometrial cancer missed, so can any of us.

I'd like to share a second story with you, because it shows a different scenario. A year ago, I was giving a talk to a group of women in New York City about taking charge of their health and the newest hormone therapy issues. A premenopausal 54-year-old woman stood up and said she had been feeling bloated and had heavy and irregular bleeding. She was concerned, but after a normal pelvic exam her doctor reassured her that she was okay, even though a pelvic exam is not sensitive enough to pick up cancer of uterus or ovaries. Then she asked me about hormone therapy. I noticed that she had a very obvious apple shape, and that she was overweight. I asked a couple of questions and found out that she had a family history of type 2 diabetes and that her mother also is apple-shaped. In addition, this woman often had irregular periods with long cycles in between, which suggests that she wasn't ovulating, and therefore she had had years of high oestrogen without the balancing progesterone. I recommended a vaginal ultrasound and endometrial biopsy, and I explained to her about her body shape and the significance of her irregular periods.

Two months later, I received an email from the woman telling me that she had been diagnosed with endometrial cancer and had just had a hysterectomy. She thanked me and said that she always knew something wasn't right, but she didn't have the right information or the proper language to discuss it. She now realises she should have been checked out months earlier, when they would have caught it at the pre-cancerous stage, and the hysterectomy wouldn't have been necessary.

Action Items for Chapter 7:
Breast and Endometrial Cancer

◆ If breast cancer runs in your immediate family, you may want to consider genetic testing to see if you carry the BRCA1 or BRCA2 gene mutations. These mutations confer a much higher risk of developing breast cancer than average. The average woman has about a 12 per cent lifetime risk of developing breast cancer; women with the BRCA1 gene mutation have a 50 to 60 per cent risk by the age of 70. Most hospitals offer genetic counselling to determine if testing is right for you. There are psychological and emotional factors to consider, in addition to possible insurance and employment ramifications. If you do not have a mutation, you can rest easier knowing that your risk is the same as every other woman's risk. If you do have a mutation, then your physician can help you do everything possible to prevent the occurrence of breast cancer or to catch it early enough to be treated successfully.

◆ All women should, if possible, have a breast exam every year or so along with a smear test. I also recommend regular breast self-exams every month, within a week after your period ends, or anytime if you are menopausal. I believe that there is no substitute for personal knowledge of your own body, and that includes your breasts. If you feel something different, or if you are concerned about changes in your breasts, speak up! And don't let anyone tell you that you are 'fine' unless he or she can prove it by biopsy or needle aspiration results.

◆ All women over age 50 should get a mammogram to check for breast cancer every year. Every woman should have a mammogram at age 40 to use as a benchmark to compare against future mammograms. I also feel that apple-shaped women who are overweight might want to consider starting yearly mammograms at age 40. If you have a strong family history of breast cancer, or if you feel that there is something wrong that doesn't show up on a mammogram, ask about a magnetic resonance imaging (MRI) scan of the breast. It tends to be more sensitive than mammograms, particularly among women with dense breasts.

◆ Stop smoking. Although not all research agrees, there are some data that suggest that smoking can increase the risk for breast cancer by up to 80 per cent. Apple-shaped women who smoke also face a greater risk of lung cancer than any other group. One study showed that women with a waist circumference larger than 100cm (39½in) had three times the risk of lung cancer compared with women with smaller waists. And it is well documented that smoking increases your stores of visceral fat! The more you smoke, the more apple-shaped you'll become and the higher your risks of all diseases, even cancer.

◆ If you have irregular or infrequent periods, talk to your doctor about progesterone therapy to prevent the unopposed oestrogen build-up of the uterine lining. If you are a postmenopausal woman and have your uterus, don't take unopposed oestrogen. Talk to your doctor about the best progesterone regimen for you.

◆ Watch for signs of endometrial cancer. This is especially true if you are an apple-shaped women and you have had irregular periods or very long cycles, if you took unopposed oestrogen, or if you didn't menstruate for years and didn't take progesterone to clean out the lining every few months. Common signs are bleeding, midcycle spotting, unusual cramping, pain with intercourse or bleeding after intercourse. Take these symptoms seriously, and do what Fran Drescher did with her final doctor – insist on proper testing, a vaginal ultrasound to measure the uterine thickness (called the 'endometrial stripe') and an endometrial biopsy.

◆ Follow the body shape programmes in Part 3 to reduce your waist measurement and thereby reduce your risks for breast and endometrial cancers.

◆ Get a good night's sleep. Studies have shown that our bodies' hormonal patterns during sleep may actually help us prevent precancerous cells from becoming cancerous. Two hormones that are affected by lack of sleep or disrupted sleep patterns are cortisol, which helps regulate the body's immune-related natural killer cells, and melatonin, which seems to have antioxidant properties and also helps regulate oestrogen production. Low levels of melatonin may also leave the cells vulnerable to DNA mutations. Women who disrupt their normal sleep cycle, by working the night shift, for example, tend to have about a 60 per cent higher risk of developing breast cancer. Women who get too little sleep may be missing out on their bodies' natural cancer-fighting abilities. Sleep is not a luxury – it's a healthy necessity!

Take to Heart ...

◆ Don't be afraid to acknowledge your shape and physical concerns to your doctor. A simple sentence can be very effective: *Doctor, I know that I carry my weight in the middle, I've had years of irregular periods or unopposed oestrogen, so I would feel better if we checked it out further.* We can't be afraid to speak up when our lives are on the line.

◆ Cancer is one of those fears that it is best to face head-on. Endometrial cancer is 100 per cent curable when it is caught early. Breast cancer is more treatable than ever, and the earlier it is caught, the better. If you feel a lump, or experience unusual vaginal bleeding or bloating, see your doctor immediately. If it is not cancer, you'll put your mind at ease. If it is cancer, then you know you got treated as early as possible.

CHAPTER 8

Osteoporosis
and Varicose Veins

Although apple-shaped women bear the brunt of most disease risk, they get a break in this chapter. Pear-shaped women have a couple of high-risk areas of their own.

The differences between visceral fat and pear-zone fat make apple-shaped women a target for the metabolic disorders, with the underlying problem residing in body chemistry – hormones, cytokines, blood glucose, lipids and sundry proteins. Their challenge is to regulate their body chemistry so that everything runs as perfectly as possible. For pear-shaped women, the underlying problem resides in structure – bones and blood vessels. Their chemistry tends to be pretty well balanced, so the challenge is to maintain the integrity of their structure so that they can remain healthy and pain free well into old age.

OSTEOPOROSIS

Osteoporosis is a disease in which bones (*osteo*) become holey or *porous*, gradually becoming thinner and weaker until they are prone to fractures. Statistics show that about 44 per cent of women aged 80 or older have osteoporosis, and another 43 per cent have enough bone loss that they can be considered to have *osteopenia,* or 'preosteoporosis'.

Most women never think about osteoporosis until it is too late. When we're young, we worry about body fat and how we look. When we're middle-aged, we also worry about how we look, but we add cancer and hot flushes to our list of major concerns. Very few women worry about the state of their bones until one day a simple slip causes a broken hip and months of recuperation and physical therapy. Or when their dentist tells them that they are about to lose their teeth because the bony part of their jaw has receded. Or, worst of all, when their vertebrae – the back bones that protect the spinal cord – start to crumble like old chalk, leaving them shorter, hump-backed and in constant severe pain.

Bones are living, growing,
and constantly changing tissues.

When you form a mental picture of bone, you probably visualise something stark and dry. Unlike blood vessels or other soft tissue body parts, bone survives long after the body has decomposed, which is why we can go to a museum and see dinosaur bones that are hundreds of millions of years old. So it surprises many women to learn that bones are not just the hardened beams of our bodies. Just as it is helpful to think of fat as adipose tissue to appreciate its function in the body, bone is known as *osseous tissue* – a term that reflects its status as an integral part of the body system. Bones are living, growing and constantly changing tissues. They are fed by blood vessels, and they communicate with the rest of the body through the nervous system and chemical messengers.

Bones have three layers. The innermost section is the soft bone marrow. That is surrounded by *trabecular bone,* sometimes called spongy bone because it has the honeycombed appearance of a sponge. The outermost layer of bone is the solid, hard cortical bone. Bony material is made up of a collagen framework shored up by cement-hard calcium phosphate. Ninety-nine per cent of the calcium in our bodies is found in our bones and teeth. But every cell in our bodies needs calcium for transmission of messages, contraction of muscle cells and other normal functions. The level of calcium in the bloodstream must remain tightly balanced for good health. Any rise or fall in the steady-state calcium level in the blood leads to severe, even life-threatening problems.

Along with acting as our physical framework, one of the functions of bone is to act as a calcium storage facility for the rest of the body. If we get enough calcium in our diets to satisfy the body's general needs, then any calcium pulled out of our bones for the blood supply will be replaced. But if we don't eat enough calcium-rich foods (or take a calcium supplement), then the body takes the calcium it needs from the bones, and it isn't replaced. Molecule by molecule, the bone loses part of its structure. Most of the calcium loss comes from the middle layer of bone – the spongy bone. As the walls of the honeycomb structure become thinner, the bone loses its integrity from the inside out. The result of this loss of bone mass is that the bone itself loses its *density.* From the outside, the bone can look strong and solid; but the inside will look like a piece of Swiss cheese, with the holes getting bigger and bigger. Obviously, the denser the bone is to begin with, the more calcium you can afford to lose before the structure becomes compromised.

If we don't eat enough calcium-rich foods (or take a calcium supplement), then the body takes the calcium it needs from the bones, and it isn't replaced.

When bones lose too much density, they become weak and are prone to break or crumble. This state is called osteoporosis. Unless you have a very astute physician, or you are a very proactive patient, you won't know you have osteoporosis until you break a bone. The most typical breaks occur either at the hip, where the long bone of the leg (the femur) is connected by a ball-and-socket joint to the pelvis, or in the back. Actually, the bones of the back don't break so much as compress – the bone loses so much structure that it eventually caves in on itself. You may also break a wrist or an ankle, depending on the kind of fall you take. Then, through a combination of X-rays and other tests, you'll be diagnosed with osteoporosis. In some cases, dentists can diagnose low bone density in the jaw. For some women, tooth loss may be their first clue that something is wrong.

Osteoporosis: The Risk Factors

Much of the risk for osteoporosis is inherited, so if your mother or either of your grandmothers had osteoporosis, you also have an increased risk. Caucasian and Asian women have the highest risks of any of the racial or ethnic groups, and African American, Latino and Hispanic women have a much lower – but still significant – risk. Small, thin women also have a very high risk, as do light-haired, blue-eyed women. Premature grey hair – being more than 50 per cent grey by the time you are 40 – has also been linked to a higher risk for osteoporosis.

At least some of the risk is due to things we do in young adulthood. Women build to their peak bone mass at age 30. That's when your bones are the densest they will ever be. After that, you either start losing bone mass, or – if you do everything right – you maintain the same amount of bone mass. You can never again rebuild bone, you can only replace the calcium that the body uses. It's sort of like stopping water from running out of a leaky bucket in the middle of a desert – you can save what's left, but you can never refill the bucket. So after age 30, everything you do goes towards protecting the bone you have. The more you abused your body by dieting when you were young, the more vigorous you'll have to be when you are older to maintain enough bone to be healthy.

One big example of bone abuse is not getting enough calcium in the teenage and young adult years. Women who had anorexia nervosa or who dieted and exercised extensively for weight control may have depleted their bone mass to dangerous levels even before they got to age 30. This is so common that doctors have called a specific group of risk factors the 'athletic triad' – disordered eating, excessive exercise and amenorrhoea (no ovulation and therefore no menstruation). In contrast to apple-shaped women or women with polycystic ovary syndrome (PCOS) who may not ovulate but continue to produce oestrogen, women with the athletic triad have very low oestrogen levels – their amenorrhoea is caused by low body weight, which disrupts a different set of hormones. This is commonly seen in teenagers, although it is increasingly being diagnosed in women in their 20s and 30s. The loss of oestrogen and progesterone causes bone loss beyond what would be expected by dieting alone.

The more you abused your body by dieting when you were young, the more vigorous you'll have to be when you are older to maintain enough bone to be healthy.

You see, oestrogen is a critical component to the replacement of calcium in bones – it is part of the equation. After menopause, when oestrogen levels plummet, bone density drops off dramatically for about 10 years before levelling off to a slower pace. Hormone therapy (HT) after menopause, which adds back the missing oestrogen, delays this bone loss. In fact, the strong positive effect on bones is one of the main benefits of HT. Many, many studies have documented that women who use hormones after menopause have better bone density than women who don't use hormones and consequently a much lower risk of fracture.

Androgens – the typically 'male' hormones – also participate in building early bone mass. Apple-shaped women, then, have the best of all worlds when it comes to their bones. They have higher levels of androgen to build bone when they are young, and they have more visceral fat to convert androgens into powerful oestrogens after menopause. They have built-in protection. That's why women with polycystic ovary syndrome (PCOS) typically have much higher bone density than women without PCOS. And studies have shown that apple-shaped women have a higher bone density than pear-shaped women.

It stands to reason, then, that most of the women who end up with osteoporosis were probably pear-shaped women when they were young. With osteoporosis, becoming apple-shaped later in life doesn't reduce your risk. Because peak bone mass occurs at age 30, whatever your body shape was in your teens and 20s will have affected your risk of developing osteoporosis 30, 40 or 50 years later.

Low body weight is also a risk factor for osteoporosis, so thin pear-shaped women will have the worst risks (especially if they are blond Caucasians or Asian). This is because body weight puts pressure on the bones, and this added force spurs more bone growth. Heavy women of all body shapes have stronger bones than thin women. This is the one time that being overweight is actually beneficial.

Sometimes being overweight is actually beneficial –
heavy women of all body shapes have stronger bones
than thin women.

I am not advocating that pear-shaped women go out and stuff themselves on pizza and cookies in the name of bone health. Although overall fat mass does improve bone density, so does overall lean mass. 'Lean mass' means muscle. The waiflike young women who prize an emaciated, non-muscled look are heading for bone trouble in the not-too-distant future. The goal should be fit and well-muscled – think of women soccer players like Mia Hamm, think of tennis players Venus and Serena Williams. (I'd like to think of an actress to emulate, but I can't. Even the ones who are fit are too underweight to be mentioned as role models.) In fact, some studies show that total lean mass contributes more to total body bone density than total fat mass in both premenopausal and postmenopausal women – so muscle is better than fat at building bone throughout the body. Apple-shaped women have the advantage here, too. Thanks again to their extra androgens, apple-shaped women naturally have greater lean muscle mass than pear-shaped women.

Strong muscles help develop strong bones.

The one place where pear-shaped women have a chance to catch up is muscle development. Studies have shown that muscle strength can affect bone density in specific body areas. For example, researchers from France studied women over age 60 for lean mass, fat mass, weight and muscle strength. They found that lean mass was respon-sible for a large portion of the bone mass, and the stronger the women's thigh muscles (quadriceps), the stronger their thigh bones. This tells us that muscle is a critical component to building and keeping bone throughout the body – and that the force exerted by specific muscle groups can help protect bone in related areas. Or, to simplify further: strong muscles help develop strong bones.

The problem is that lean muscle mass naturally decreases as we get older, in part because of physiologic factors, and in part because we are generally less physically active. Pear-shaped women have an uphill battle from the beginning – they start out with lower bone density, they have less lean muscle mass and they have less natural oestrogen after menopause. By the time they reach their 70s or 80s, some pear-shaped women are walking around on bones that are little better than hollow egg shells. One false step and they could crumble.

Testing for Osteoporosis

Women who have an increased risk for osteoporosis are usually advised by their doctors to have a special test called dual-energy x-ray absorptiometry (DXA or DEXA). This simple, painless scan, which takes between 10 and 30 minutes, uses low-dose radiation to measure bone density. The result is given in the form of two scores:

1. T score, which compares your bones to the bones of a young, healthy woman at peak bone mass. A score above −1 is considered 'normal'. A score between −1 and −2.5 is considered at risk, and you may hear the word 'osteopenia', which basically means low bone density but not at osteoporosis severity. A score below −2.5 is considered the cutoff for defining osteoporosis. For every decrease by a score of −1, the risk of fractures doubles.

2. Z score, which compares your bones to the bones of someone of your same age.

It is quite possible that your T score could indicate that you have osteoporosis, while your Z score is relatively normal. If most women your age have osteoporosis, and you have osteoporosis, then you will have similar bone density to most women your age. This is why you should be most concerned with your T score – how you compare with *optimal* bone density. The Z score is mostly helpful to doctors. For example, if a young woman has a Z score that is much lower than similar women her age, she may have a secondary cause of osteoporosis, such as an eating disorder. When I was the medical director at the Center for Women's Health in Philadelphia I saw the lowest and most disturbing bone densities in young women with anorexia.

I recommend that all pear-shaped women get a DXA scan to use as a baseline as they approach menopause. This tells them what their peak bone mass is before menopause, before they suffer the rapid bone loss from lower oestrogen levels. Apple-shaped women should be tested by age 65. By then, even if they had high bone mass at age 30, ageing naturally will have caused gradual bone loss.

Remember, this is a baseline measurement, a snapshot of where you are now. Many women in their late 40s panic if their T score shows that they have osteopenia. I tell them that it doesn't necessarily mean they are currently losing bone, just that they didn't build up a strong bone density in their youth. Further losses can be prevented. Just do everything right, have the DXA repeated in a year to see if you have lost any additional bone. If not, then you know that you've made a difference. If you have lost bone in that year, then the doctor will check for other factors that might contribute to bone loss, such as an overactive thyroid.

Osteoporosis Prevention

Ideally, we should all be practising osteoporosis prevention throughout our lives. Children are taught good dental hygiene with the promise that it will keep their teeth from rotting and falling out when they are older. Long-term bone health is just as critical in the childhood through young adult years.

If you are a woman younger than age 30, now is the time to take advantage of your body's ability to increase bone density. If you are over age 30, then your job is to protect the bone you have, and try to make calcium replacement as efficient as possible. The best ways to accomplish these tasks are:

◆ Get plenty of calcium in your diet. Foods that are high in calcium include milk, yoghurt, cheese, tofu, broccoli, pak choi, mustard greens, cauliflower, legumes and almonds. Still, most people don't get all the calcium they need from food alone, so I always recommended taking a calcium supplement just to be sure. (See the diet sections in Part 3 for specific recommendations by body type.)

◆ Get vitamin D. Calcium and vitamin D work as partners in creating bone. Neither one can work without the other. Vitamin D is made naturally in the skin in response to sunlight. All you need is the equivalent of about 15 minutes of sunlight on the skin of your arms every day to make the vitamin D you need. Unfortunately, with extended work schedules and the (wise) use of sunscreen, many people don't get even that limited amount of sunlight every day. In that case, be sure to take a multivitamin that contains at least 400 IU of vitamin D.

◆ Eat a diet rich in all kinds of fruits and vegetables. There's more to bone health than just calcium. Fruits and vegetables contain high amounts of other vitamins and minerals that contribute to bone strength, including iron, zinc, magnesium, potassium and vitamin C.

◆ Avoid fried foods and store-bought baked goods. Bone loss seems to be greater among women who eat larger amounts of certain kinds of fats – especially the kinds of fats used to make fried foods (including chips and potato crisps) and packaged biscuits, breads, cakes and other snack treats.

◆ If you drink alcohol, do so in moderation. One glass of alcohol per day has been associated with *less* bone loss in the spine . . . but more than that increases bone loss. If you don't drink alcohol, don't start. It does not help that much. But if you enjoy a glass of wine with dinner, you won't be hurting your bones to continue – as long as you don't drink the whole bottle.

◆ Stop smoking – it decreases bone mass.

◆ Do weight-bearing or resistance exercise. Exercises that put stress on the bones of the body help preserve bone density. It's almost as if the bones sense that they need to be stronger to hold up the extra weight, so they respond by becoming denser. The best general exercises for building bone are walking (but not running or jogging), dancing, aerobics, cycling and gardening. The worst exercise for building bone is swimming because the water supports your weight, so your bones are not stressed at all. Even better are resistance-training exercises, as described in chapter 13. Studies have shown that resistance training helps reduce age-related bone loss and can actually help increase bone density. Researchers found that postmenopausal women who did resistance training just two days per week for a year gained 1.0 per cent bone mass in their thigh and back bones, while women who did no training lost 2.5 per cent of their bone mass in those same locations.

◆ If you are a pear-shaped woman, talk with your doctor about whether taking HT after menopause might be a good way for you to prevent osteoporosis. The issue of HT is complex, and it is not right for everyone (see chapter 4 for more information).

You may have heard that caffeine reduces bone mass, and many postmenopausal women reluctantly gave up their coffee and tea for the sake of their bones. Some early studies did show a relationship, usually when measuring the amount of calcium excreted in the urine. Upon further research, it turned out that the body has a better balancing system than we thought, so that any calcium loss was made up by extra calcium retention later in the day. Plus, some of the early studies were faulty. Many coffee drinkers are also smokers, and smoking causes bone loss. In the studies, it looked like coffee was the bad guy when really it was the cigarettes. Later studies that looked specifically at the effects on bones confirmed that drinking caffeine-containing beverages does *not* increase the risk of osteoporosis or bone loss. The only group that had any negative effects were elderly white women, who had a slight decrease in bone density in their thigh bones. In other words, if you are generally healthy and get plenty of calcium in your diet, there is no evidence that drinking coffee or tea will hurt your bones.

The issue of carbonated beverages is also controversial. Studies of children found that those who drink large amounts of fizzy drinks (which are usually sweet) are more likely to get bone fractures. But researchers now think that it isn't the fizzy drink itself that caused the bone loss. By choosing to drink fizzy drinks instead of milk, the children simply weren't getting enough calcium to keep their bones strong. There have been very few studies on adults, and those show little or no bad effects from soft drinks. For example, a study published in a 2001 issue of the *American Journal of Clinical Nutrition* showed that fizzy drinks did not cause calcium to leach from the body (as had been previously reported). And an earlier study from researchers at Brigham and Women's Hospital in Boston showed that over an intensive eight-week study, fizzy drinks did not have a bad effect on urine or blood levels of calcium.

So with everything else you have to worry about, take caffeine and fizzy drinks off your list. *However,* I would like to go on record as recommending that women of all ages reduce the amount of fizzy drinks they consume – both sugared and artificially sweetened. Sugared drinks add unnecessary calories without adding any vitamins or minerals. Artificial sweeteners are controversial, and I come down on the side of avoidance. I believe that we don't know the last word on the safety of artificial sweeteners. We thought that artificial fats – the trans fats – were healthy until we discovered that they are a major contributor to heart disease. Some women have reported headaches, seizures or mood swings after drinking diet fizzy drinks, which tells me that they have some sort of effect in the brain. I personally avoid any artificially sweetened food or drink.

Other Osteoporosis Considerations

Many women don't know that some medications they may be taking might be weakening their bones. For example, a large number of women are currently taking levothyroxine for hypothyroidism. But having too much thyroid hormone can weaken bones. If the dosage is not properly adjusted and regularly monitored, bone loss can occur. Also, the common seizure medication Dilantin (phenytoin) causes bone thinning by interfering with the synthesis and metabolism of vitamin D. Steroids taken for a long time, such as for control of asthma, can cause major loss of calcium and bone loss.

Osteoporosis is not inevitable – there is always something that can be done. Start, of course, with diet and exercise changes in chapters 11, 12 and 13. Pear-shaped women just entering menopause should talk with their doctors about HT. Women with osteopoenia might want to talk with their doctors about taking a thiazide diuretic, especially if they have high blood pressure. Although most women take this medication for hypertension, studies have shown that it can reduce fracture risk 22 to 37 per cent, with the medication seeming to become more effective with longer use. After considering hormone therapy, this is always my next recommendation for treatment.

The final course of action – if all the above methods fail – is to use a potent bone-building drug, such as Fosamax (alendronate) or Actonel (risedronate). These drugs have been demonstrated to slow or entirely stop bone loss and reduce the risk of fracture by half.

A note of caution: many doctors are choosing to prescribe Evista instead of putting patients on HT. Evista is from the class of drugs known in the United States as Selective Oestrogen Receptor Modulators – the same class of drugs as tamoxifen, which is used to treat breast cancer. I don't believe that we have enough information to know the long-term safety of SERMs. For example, we know that tamoxifen is only safe for five years, after which, its effects *reverse*. I caution women who are otherwise healthy not to be so quick to take Evista for osteoporosis. HT has a much longer track record, and is very effective in preventing bone loss, even in small doses.

Marcy's and Samantha's Stories

I like to consider Marcy a success story because she wasn't afraid to take action to keep herself healthy. She ate a healthy diet, and exercised whenever her busy schedule would allow, so she had a good head start. But Marcy was also pear-shaped and slender, with blond hair and blue eyes – the perfect combination for osteoporosis. When she turned 50, she got a baseline DXA. We found that her T score was -1.8 for her spine, and -1.4 for her hips. This means that she did have some bone loss at baseline, most likely from hereditary factors. She didn't panic. Instead, she began taking calcium and vitamin D supplements and started doing more resistance-training exercises than before. When she started going through menopause, she decided to take HT. She repeated the DXA every year. After menopause, most women lose up to 5 per cent of their bone mass yearly for the first five years. But Marcy's DXA has remained exactly the same for the past four years. She was able to maintain her bone mass with this simple regimen.

Samantha had a more severe situation. As a young woman, Samantha had had an eating disorder, and she continued to 'watch her weight closely' as an adult. At age 45, she had a minor fall while ice skating and broke her wrist. Although she was young, it didn't seem right, so I sent her to get a DXA to see if she had premature bone loss. Sure enough, her T score was -2.6 at her spine, and -2.0 at her hips. When I questioned her further, it turned out that she was also currently taking diet pills that contained thyroid hormone. I checked her thyroid hormone blood levels and found that she had levels that were way too high, making her hyperthyroid, which means that she was losing huge amounts of bone. I got her to stop taking diet pills, started her on calcium and vitamin D supplements, and got her to commit to doing resistance exercises. Because her bones had such low density, she also chose to take Fosamax to prevent further fractures. My hope will be that as she approaches menopause she can stop the medication, continue the lifestyle changes and perhaps begin taking low-dose oestrogen.

Different women, different levels of bone loss, different problems. And yet, they are both managing their bone health well. Fortunately, osteoporosis is not immediately life threatening. If you pay attention, get regular DXA scans, and prevent further bone loss through lifestyle and medication, you should be able to have a sturdy skeleton for the rest of your life.

VARICOSE VEINS

Ever wonder why blood doesn't pool in your feet? We know that the heart pumps to circulate blood throughout the body, but it's a long way from the feet back up to the heart. Actually, there are tiny flaps or valves in veins that open to allow blood to surge forward, but then close to keep the blood from falling backward. If these valves become damaged or weak, some blood can leak backward, and eventually the vein becomes congested and can start to bulge. That's what varicose veins are – the enlarged, cordlike veins, usually in the legs, that don't move blood forward efficiently. If this happens in a tiny vein that is closer to the surface of the skin, the result is called 'spider veins'. These look like finely etched blue, purple or red markings, as if someone drew on the skin with a coloured pen.

In the Western world generally, between 20 and 30 per cent of women have varicose veins (as compared with about 2 per cent in rural India, for example). They are caused in part by hereditary factors, so if your mother has them, then they are another gift from her to you. Hormones also help cause varicose veins. Women are more likely to see them appear during puberty, at menopause and if they take oral contraceptives or HT. The most common time for varicose veins to appear is during pregnancy, when you get the one-two-three punch of high hormone levels, extra pressure on veins from an enlarged uterus, and a greater volume of blood to pump throughout the body. Other factors that weaken blood vessels and contribute to developing varicose veins are exposure to sunlight, prolonged sitting or standing and obesity.

Of course, body shape also contributes, but probably for many of the same reasons already listed. We know from research that apple-shaped women have about a 20 per cent lower risk of varicose veins than pear-shaped women. However, we don't really know why. Researchers have suggested that it's because pear-shaped women carry extra weight in their legs, which equates to more pressure on leg veins. Alternatively, because a pear shape is inherited, it could be that varicose veins are simply tied into the genetic package – inherit the thighs, inherit the veins. It has also been posited that pear-shaped women tend to have a defect in their lymphatic system. This is a little-known system in the body that functions similarly to the circulatory system, except instead of moving blood around the body, it moves lymphatic fluid. The lymphatic system has two roles – it is involved in immune function, and it collects fluid and plasma proteins that leak from the blood and returns them to the bloodstream. If the lymphatic system doesn't work well, then that leaked fluid will collect in the body tissues, where it can cause general puffiness from oedema. That tissue swelling puts pressure on the blood vessels, and varicose veins can result.

Varicose veins can be purely a cosmetic problem, or they can cause chronic aching, discomfort and a sense of heaviness, particularly after standing for long periods of time. Moving around will usually help alleviate the ache because it gets the blood moving again. If large varicose veins become severe, the congestion may become so bad that blood is no longer circulated properly. This condition is called venous insufficiency, and it can cause a life-threatening blood clot (deep vein thrombosis). This isn't something that will happen by surprise – you will usually feel considerable discomfort in your legs, and the veins may become swollen, warm, red or painful to touch. If you develop these symptoms, see your doctor.

Preventing Varicose Veins

You won't be able to prevent varicose veins entirely. If you have a predisposition to developing spider veins, they will appear as sure as hair turns grey with age. However, there are things you can do to help reduce their number and severity:

◆ Consider specially designed maternity support tights while pregnant. These are uncomfortable to wear in the summer, and they can be a real bother to put on (I wore them during my pregnancies), but they prevent your legs from swelling and aching. They have gradient compression, so the pressure is highest at the ankle and lightest up at the thigh. Among the leading brands are Aristoc and Marks & Spencer. Talk with your obstetrician about whether support stockings might be good for you.

◆ Try not to stand or sit in one place for very long without moving. Take small breaks to walk about, or shift your weight from one leg to another. If you are sitting, do not cross your legs at the knee – this puts extra pressure on delicate veins.

◆ When resting, try to elevate your legs. Prop them up with pillows, lie across the couch, or commandeer the recliner.

◆ Reduce water retention in your legs by eliminating excess salt from your diet. Take the salt shaker off the table and avoid foods with too much added sodium.

◆ Avoid too much sunlight on your legs, and because fair-skinned women can develop spider veins around their noses, always wear sunscreen on your face.

Varicose Vein Treatments

For large varicose veins, surgery may be necessary to remove the damaged vein from the leg. Smaller varicose veins and spider veins are most often and most easily treated with sclerotherapy, in which a special solution is injected into the vein to close it off. The vein dies, turns into scar tissue, and fades. This is obviously only done in relatively small veins. This simple procedure, which is usually done right in the doctor's consulting room without anaesthesia, has about a 50 to 90 per cent success rate. More recently, laser surgery has been perfected for use on the face and the legs. There are no needles, just a beam of laser light that damages the vein so that it disappears. If your varicose veins bother you, ask your doctor which type of treatment might be best. It's important to note, however, that treatment for cosmetic purposes will probably need to be done privately. And of course, getting rid of some spider veins won't guarantee clear legs – chances are that others will appear within a few years.

Action Items for Chapter 8:
Osteoporosis and Varicose Veins

◆ If you have not yet gone through menopause but are not having periods, that is called *amenorrhoea,* and it should be checked out by a physician. There are a number of possible causes, but the net result could mean an increased risk of osteoporosis. You may need to take oral contraceptives to balance out your hormones.

◆ Get a DXA scan *if:* you are a pear-shaped women over age 40; you are over age 50 and had a bone fracture; you had an eating disorder as a young woman; or you are taking thyroid medication, long-term steroid medication or the anti-epileptic drug phenytoin.

◆ If you have osteopoenia or osteoporosis, get a repeat DXA every year or two to make sure that you are maintaining the bone you have. If your DXA is normal, repeat the test every five years. You will probably need to have this, too, done privately. Please don't let that be a deterrent to getting the test. Isn't your health worth it?

◆ Pear-shaped women who take HT or oral contraceptives need to be aware that their vein problems may slightly increase their risk of blood clots. Always tell your doctor if you start to feel a throbbing, achy discomfort along with swelling or tightness in one leg. (Usually only one leg is affected by clots, so if both legs ache or swell, something else is going on.) If you need surgery, make sure you stop taking the pill or hormones two weeks beforehand to prevent blood clots. You'll also need to temporarily stop taking them if you are immobilised for a while, such as if you are put in a leg cast or require prolonged hospitalisation or bed rest. And, of course, if you ever develop a blood clot while on hormones, you must stop taking them and can consider them unsafe for you forever.

Take to Heart . . .

◆ Some women who find themselves facing low bone density feel guilty for not exercising more, not taking vitamins or not seeing their doctor sooner. These kinds of regrets are understandable, but they aren't productive. There's no sense in beating yourself up over something you did or didn't do in the past. If osteoporosis is a concern, take action and move forward. Don't ruminate over past decisions. There's not a teenage girl alive who plans her meals around her risk of developing osteoporosis after age 50. You are not to blame for the ravages of time.

CHAPTER 9

Stress, Anger and Depression

A lthough we conceive them to be purely mental phenomena, emotions are also physical events. We understand and identify them from the way they affect our bodies – we can have aching hearts, gnawed stomachs, raw nerves and burned-out brains. Even the language we use to describe how we feel is created from physical images: anger builds up, sadness settles in, stress hits us. This is because every emotion is associated with very specific biochemical reactions that have repercussions throughout the body.

Brain nerves (*neurons*) communicate with each other through a combination of chemical and electrical signals. Every thought causes an electrical impulse to run through a group of neurons. When the impulse reaches the nerve endings, it triggers the release of tiny amounts of chemical messengers called *neurotransmitters,* which flood into the tiny gap (*synapse*) between the original nerve and the receiving nerve. If enough neurotransmitter reaches the receiving nerve, it causes an electrical impulse to begin in that nerve, and the process continues. With this method, each neuron can communicate directly with potentially dozens of other neurons, and each of those may com- municate in turn with dozens more. And it all occurs in the tiniest sliver of a split second. In the time it takes you to *think* about scratching your nose, millions of brain cells have received the message and you will have visualised yourself scratching your nose even before you move a muscle. If you actually decide to scratch your nose, a new communication among neurons takes place, and your brain will signal your arm to lift, your hand to extend and your finger to scratch. No matter how quickly you try to act, your brain cells can always keep up, spreading the messages of your thoughts and intentions almost instantaneously.

Your neurons fire not only in response to your thoughts and intentions, but also in response to signals from the body. The nervous system connects every body part, every organ, every square centimetre of skin to your brain. If you stub your toe, your brain receives the message of pain in less than a second. In response it sends signals to other parts of the body so they can respond appropriately – for example, inflammatory chemicals called cytokines will rush to initiate healing, making the toe swollen, red and painful. The brain also responds to more subtle signals from the body. If you run short of energy and it is time to eat, your brain will receive messages from a number of different sources as your stomach feels empty, your blood glucose level drops and your level of insulin and other hormones falls. Your brain will coordinate and translate all those clues, and label the sensation as 'hunger'.

The body and mind are mutually influenced.

So brain chemistry can change in response to your thoughts or in response to signals from the body. Emotions also cause brain chemistry changes . . . and changes in brain chemistry can cause emotion. It is a complex interweaving of thoughts and physical signals, and many times it is impossible to know how an emotion began. For example, the neurotransmitter called serotonin is associated with a general sense of well-being. In scientific experiments, when researchers inhibit the synthesis of serotonin, people who receive that treatment feel and act depressed. Conversely, when depressed people are given Prozac or other medications that increase the amount of serotonin available to neurons, they usually feel happier. But which came first, the depression or the low amounts of serotonin? In the real world outside of the laboratory, when brain chemicals respond at the speed of thought, it is difficult to know for certain. The most likely scenario is that body and mind are mutually influenced – that what we think and feel affects our physical selves, and in response our bodies create a chemical environment that makes us more or less likely to experience particular emotions.

THE MIND-BODY CONNECTION

As individuals, we are each a unique combination of mind and body – thoughts and emotions and flesh and blood woven into an intricate biological tapestry. The power of our minds to affect our physical selves has been recognised since the time of Galen, around A.D. 170, who listed 'passions or perturbations of the soul' among the factors that can upset the balance of health. Our thoughts and emotions have such strong effects on the body that we are quite capable of making ourselves ill. The so-called psychosomatic diseases are not 'all in the head', as they are frequently believed to be – they are very real diseases that can be quite debilitating. These conditions include irritable bowel syndrome, chronic fatigue syndrome, fibromyalgia, insomnia and many cases of unexplainable pain or fatigue. They often have their origins in physical reactions to psychological processes and end up causing pain, exhaustion and distress.

But really, if you dig deep enough, most diseases can be seen as having a mind-body connection. Almost every disorder can be made worse by strong negative emotions. People who have autoimmune diseases, such as multiple sclerosis or systemic lupus erythematosus, notice that their symptoms flare up when they are under stress. Stress has been linked to type 2 diabetes, the metabolic syndrome and cardiovascular disease. It can induce rashes, asthma attacks, back spasms, headaches and allergic reactions. If you have any pain, stress makes it hurt more, and if you run into any virus or bacteria, stress makes you more susceptible to their effects.

We also know that stress is closely allied with depression and anger. In fact, depression, anxiety and hostility are often considered components of stress. It came as no surprise, therefore, when a 2004 report from the Women's Health Initiative stated that depression increases the risk of heart disease by about 50 per cent in postmenopausal women. Anger and hostility have also been strongly linked to heart disease. Other studies have demonstrated that depression can increase the risk of type 2 diabetes by up to 63 per cent.

Almost every disorder can be made worse by strong negative emotions.

Much of this mind-body connection can be traced to the effects of powerful emotions on the hypothalamic-pituitary-adrenocortical (HPA) axis. The HPA axis is a potent feedback loop that involves three different areas of the body: a brain structure called the hypothalamus; the pituitary gland, located in the brain; and the adrenal cortex, located above the kidneys. These three organs communicate with each other through chemical messengers, each signalling others to start or stop making various hormones.

Once the HPA axis is activated, it produces two main effects. First, HPA axis activation causes the body to secrete large quantities of a hormone called cortisol. Cortisol has several effects in the body, including increasing blood glucose levels and blood pressure, creating insulin resistance and causing the deposition of visceral fat. In fact, cortisol is generally recognised as one of the main hormones involved in regulating body fat distribution. Excess cortisol means more visceral fat and an apple shape. Second, HPA axis activation causes an increase in the production of the male hormones known as androgens, but only in women. By now I'm sure you understand that more androgens means more visceral fat and less pear-zone fat. So if we have long-term or frequent HPA axis activation, the result will be more visceral fat due to the excess production of cortisol and androgens.

There are many different physiologic reasons why the HPA axis might be activated, but the most common causes are stress, anger and depression. Knowing that HPA axis activation causes increased visceral fat, scientists have been investigating some of the relationships among these emotional states and body shape. The results have been eye-opening.

STRESS

One of the major factors that causes HPA axis activation is stress. When the mind and body feel stressed, the HPA axis goes into overdrive, signalling the cascade of events that results in lots of cortisol being dumped into the bloodstream. In fact, cortisol is the main hormone involved in stress – when scientists want to objectively measure the effects of stress, they measure cortisol levels in the blood or saliva.

To make matters worse, stress also triggers our fight-or-flight response. The human body tries to maintain a relatively steady and balanced internal environment, but when we perceive that we are threatened, we can go into a state of high alert. Our brain sends out signals that scream *Code Red. Prepare for danger. Get ready to run. RUN!* The body responds. It pours glucose into the bloodstream for quick energy (partly through the actions of cortisol), it shoots out adrenaline, our hearts race, blood pressure rises, and we are ready to escape the horrible threat. In modern times, however, the danger is usually something relatively innocuous, such as getting reprimanded by the boss, having to do the school run on the same day you have a dentist appointment or having the in-laws call to say they are coming to visit for a week. All that urgent body preparation has no outlet. We cannot run, because the stress is inside us – our own fear, time pressure and sense of distress. If we could run, we would use up that extra glucose in our blood. But we can't, so it stays there; insulin rises and visceral fat starts to accumulate.

Pear-shaped women who experience chronic stress are likely to turn into apple-shaped women. And apple-shaped women who experience chronic stress are more likely to develop the metabolic syndrome, type 2 diabetes and heart disease.

For all women, stress mixes a Molotov cocktail of hormones, a dangerous combination of visceral fat-creating cortisol *and* visceral fat-creating androgens. Pear-shaped women who experience chronic stress are likely to turn into apple-shaped women. And apple-shaped women who experience chronic stress are more likely to develop the metabolic syndrome, type 2 diabetes and heart disease.

Stress and Body Shape

But all women are not created equal when it comes to stress. When researchers measured the specific effects of stress, they found that apple-shaped women have a hypersensitivity or overreactivity when it comes to general HPA axis regulation. Basically, their HPA axis is on a hair trigger, likely to shoot off at the slightest provocation. And when their HPA axis is activated, apple-shaped women produce higher levels of cortisol than pear-shaped women – and the larger the waist, the larger the amount of cortisol secreted. Even when they are sleeping, apple-shaped women secrete more cortisol than pear-shaped women, so it is not merely a question of psychology. There is a fundamental physical difference that causes more cortisol, which means more visceral fat.

And yet, we can't ignore the psychology. Apple-shaped women also exhibit more outward signs of psychological distress than pear-shaped women. During stress experiments, apple-shaped women report feeling more threatened by the laboratory tests, perform more poorly and describe themselves as having more stress than pear-shaped women. So stress really does hit apple-shaped women harder than pear-shaped women, leading to more subjective feelings of discomfort, as well as worse objective measures in the form of task performance deficits and higher cortisol levels. Interestingly, lean apple-shaped women in this study were even more vulnerable to stress than overweight apple-shaped women. Over the course of several days of testing and stress, the overweight apple-shaped women seemed to adapt, and their cortisol levels didn't rise as high by the end of the experiment. The lean apple-shaped women never got used to it – their cortisol levels remained high day after day.

Stress and Disease

Overreactivity to stress is more worrisome than many women know. If stress continues over a significant period of time so that the secretion of cortisol is continuously high, the adrenal glands can become depleted. If stress continues or a new stressor appears, the body will send signals asking for more cortisol, but the adrenal glands will have run dry. When this happens, health suffers. A person can feel fatigue or have a total physical collapse. Some researchers believe that HPA axis hypersensitivity and later adrenal insufficiency may play a part in the development of type 2 diabetes, fibromyalgia and chronic fatigue syndrome. We already know that apple-shaped women have a much higher risk for type 2 diabetes, so this connection makes intuitive sense. I don't know of any studies that have looked at body shape in relation to fibromyalgia, and only a few have investigated body fat's connection to chronic fatigue syndrome. Still, it wouldn't surprise me if future research showed that apple-shaped women had a greater risk for those diseases, too.

There is some evidence that this might be true. A study by researchers in Belgium found that people with chronic fatigue syndrome had significantly more visceral fat than people without chronic fatigue syndrome. Another study, this one conducted by researchers at Harvard Medical School, found that women with chronic fatigue syndrome were more likely to have a history of polycystic ovary syndrome (PCOS) than women without chronic fatigue syndrome. Because women with PCOS are the extreme model for apple-shaped women, it is likely that there is a very real connection between body shape and chronic fatigue.

If we look at measures other than cortisol, we see that stress also causes an increase in inflammation, as noted by higher levels of C-reactive protein (CRP) and interleukin-6 (IL-6). As reported in chapter 6, inflammation has a strong link to heart disease. Because proinflammatory chemicals are secreted by visceral fat, apple-shaped women already have more inflammation than pear-shaped women.

When we experience stress, everything goes up – cortisol levels, inflammation, adrenaline, blood glucose and blood pressure. It's easy to see how stress pushes apple-shaped women even faster into the metabolic syndrome, diabetes and heart disease. And don't forget that stress also contributes to waist size. Over the long run, we would expect to see stressed-out women having higher waist-to-hip ratios (WHR) than calmer women, *and* stressed-out, apple-shaped women should have higher rates of disease. Studies seem to bear that theory out. For example, we know that apple-shaped women have much higher rates of type 2 diabetes than pear-shaped women. If you take a group of women with type 2 diabetes, the ones who are more stressed, angry or depressed will tend to have higher WHRs. The chain of logic suggests that their passionate and frequent emotions caused so much cortisol and androgen release that their waists grew larger and larger over the years, making them the most appley of the apple-shaped women.

ANGER

Back in the 1970s, scientists discovered that some people had what they called the 'Type A' personality. These were defined at the time as hard-driving, ambitious, tense, high-strung, worried, easily angered people who, because of the mind-body effects of these personality characteristics, were thought to have a higher risk of heart disease. Later research refined the concept of Type A, and it was discovered that of all those personality factors, only anger and hostility were related to heart disease. Now it is believed that anger exerts these effects by triggering the HPA axis, leading to the same cascade of hormones that stress causes.

Anger and Body Shape

Given that apple-shaped women have a more reactive HPA axis, scientists have speculated that these women would be more sensitive to anger than pear-shaped women. It seems to be true. The Healthy Women Study followed a group of more than 475 middle-aged women for more than a decade. The researchers discovered that apple-shaped women generally had higher levels of anger, anxiety and depression than pear-shaped women, and that the level of distress increased as waist circumference increased. As the researchers took measurements throughout the decade, they found that the women who had the greatest increases in anger scores also had the highest increases in amounts of visceral fat, regardless of how much weight they gained overall.

This is a great example of the chicken-or-the-egg sequence quandary. Were the women angry and depressed because they were gaining weight, or was their anger and depression fuelling their weight gain? In this case, there was at least a partial answer. In a follow-up analysis, the researchers discovered that women who were generally angry at the beginning of the study, when they were at their thinnest, had a nearly 50 per cent higher risk of developing the metabolic syndrome by the end of the study. And the angrier the women became over the years, the greater their chances of developing the metabolic syndrome. So the emotions came first, and the weight gain and disease came later. Considering that waist circumference is one of the possible criteria for diagnosing the metabolic syndrome, it is likely that these women were mostly apple-shaped. The researchers did a similar study, but this time testing children, who are typically not as weight conscious as adult women. They measured the children's general level of hostility, then followed them for three years. The kids who had the highest levels of hostility at the beginning of the study were more likely to have the metabolic syndrome three years later! Again, emotions led to disease.

Another study followed a group of 374 young men and women to see which personality traits might contribute to heart disease. At the beginning of the study, researchers assessed lifestyle, demographic and physiologic variables, and also measured various personality traits of the subjects, including hostility. After 10 years, the participants had computed tomography (CT) scans to look at the amount of calcification they had in their arteries, a measure that determines heart disease risk. People who had high hostility levels were almost 10 times more likely to have a significant amount of artery calcification compared with nonhostile people.

If you are angry, you run a greater risk
of becoming apple-shaped in the future.

So it seems that being generally angry and hostile leads to a change in body chemistry that helps create an apple-shaped body, which in turn is associated with a higher disease risk. This is not to say that all apple-shaped women are angry or hostile – but if you are angry, you run a greater risk of becoming apple-shaped in the future. And if you are angry and already apple-shaped, you will likely increase your waist size without really doing anything very different from anyone else, because your emotions will lay down fat for you. When anger activates the HPA axis, the results are the same, whether you are an adult or a child, man or woman – excess cortisol sets you up for increased visceral fat and all the diseases associated with it. For women, though, the results are even more devastating, because of the additional androgens created.

Anger is a tough subject for many women. In most societies, including our own, it is still considered inappropriate and/or unattractive for women to express anger. We don't want to be seen as uncooperative, unkind, nasty, explosive or hostile. That doesn't mean we don't feel anger – we just don't express it. But as with stress, sublimated anger still activates the HPA axis. For many women, anger is a response to frustration, isolation or a sense of helplessness. There are no easy ways to avoid situations that make us feel that way. The trick is to find different ways to cope with angry feelings, and to adopt a less volatile attitude. As angry as the world can make us, it is an unproductive emotion. Nothing gets done better, easier or faster when we are angry. Worse, it can set you up for a lifetime of disease. Women with an explosive personality are doing themselves more harm than they think.

DEPRESSION

Many psychologists say that depression is simply anger turned inward. Whether or not that is true, anger and depression do have similar effects. They both activate the HPA axis, they both cause increased cortisol levels and they both are related to an increased risk of heart disease. Some scientists believe that depression may be triggered by chronic stress, which also makes sense. Studies have shown that people who have been diagnosed with major depression have higher levels of cortisol than nondepressed people. Even young children who are depressed have higher cortisol levels. And when children are presented with a frustrating task, the cortisol levels of depressed children went up much higher than those of nondepressed children, showing that they react with greater sensitivity and higher levels of distress much the same way as apple-shaped women.

Depression and Body Shape

Given that depressed people have higher cortisol levels, you might assume that they would also be more inclined to be apple-shaped. You would be correct. Studies that have used CT scans to measure the amount of visceral fat in depressed and nondepressed women show that women who are depressed have about twice as much abdominal fat as women who are not depressed – and the greater the amount of cortisol, the more visceral fat. This means that women who are depressed are more likely to be apple-shaped. Again, let me stress that not all apple-shaped women are depressed, but being apple-shaped may be a risk factor for becoming depressed.

EMOTIONS

The connection among all these psychological factors – stress, anger and depression – is cortisol. And apple-shaped women are chock-full of it. With their hypersensitive, hyperreactive HPA axis, they are likely to have more cortisol in their bodies at any given time. Under stress, they become more distressed – most likely because of the physiologic effects of the HPA axis activation, not because they are 'weak' or 'babyish' – and their cortisol levels soar higher than those of pear-shaped women under similar stress. More cortisol equals more abdominal fat. Similarly, women who are depressed or angry are also more likely to be apple-shaped. Of course, it is possible that excess visceral fat may also have some effect on the dysregulation of the HPA axis. Visceral fat is an endocrine gland, and it may be part of the feedback loop that regulates and balances the HPA axis. This would mean that adding weight in the apple zone could lead to further hyperreactivity of the HPA axis, which would mean still more added weight in the apple zone, and so on.

Breaking the Cycle of Weight Gain and Emotions

In theory, if you break one link in the chain, you can break the cycle.

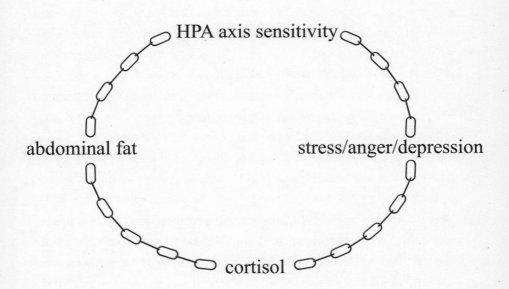

The easiest link to attack, because it is the one you have the most control over, is abdominal fat. Losing centimetres here will not only help you avoid heart disease and diabetes, it may also help you fight depression and reduce your stress reactions. If visceral adipose tissue has feedback systems that affect cortisol production or secretion – and it very well may – then reducing the amount of fat around your middle may make you feel better mentally as well as physically. The best way to lose girth is to follow the programme for apple-shaped women in Part 3 of this book.

Losing centimetres here will not only help you avoid heart disease and diabetes, it may also help you fight depression and reduce your stress reactions.

The next easiest link to attack is emotions. How do you stop stress or anger from taking over your body? The answer is relatively simple: eliminate stress and anger. I'm not being flip – I'm asking you to consider a massive change of attitude. Ask any researcher in the field what defines psychological stress, and you'll hear the same answer: *you* do. If you think something is stressful, then it is – to you. The same is true of anger. It all depends on how we respond to it. Some people react to very minor events as though the world were about to cave in. Other people can find the bright side to just about any situation.

Perfect example: a woman I know moved into her newly built house on a Monday, and that Friday a plumbing error caused the sewer to back up into her house through the basement toilet. Sewer water, faeces and filth spewed over half the basement. Biohazard clean-up teams had to rip out the brand-new carpeting and disinfect the concrete floor underneath. Portions of the walls had to be removed and replaced. Wooden studs had to be specially treated for bacteria and mould. And yet, this woman was remarkably calm. Neighbours, drawn by the commotion of the work crews, commented on how oddly serene she seemed as she sat on her front porch reading, waiting for the biohazard team to finish its work. When she told this story two years later, the event became an adventure with a happy ending. 'One set of neighbours gave us a key to their house so we would have a clean place to live,' she said. 'Another gave us a gift certificate to a local restaurant. If it weren't for the sewer blowing up, I would never have known what a warm and welcoming neighbourhood we had moved into!' I don't know if it is a coincidence, but this woman is pear-shaped.

The answer really may be as simple as changing your outlook. Researchers have discovered that people secrete cortisol in response to large stresses, and also to routine daily hassles such as getting caught in traffic or burning the toast. In addition, cortisol levels go up when people remember past stress, or when they anticipate future stress! So it's not enough that we are gaining visceral fat because of our stressful lives, we are making ourselves apple-shaped simply by *imagining* stress. The key component, however, was that the cortisol concentrations went up *only when the individuals felt angry, stressed or distressed* about the events. If they didn't have an emotional reaction, or when they controlled their emotional reaction, then cortisol levels stayed balanced.

We can make ourselves apple-shaped
simply by *imagining* stress.

I'm not talking about bottling up your anger or stress – your body can't be fooled so easily. *Feeling* stress is what counts, not whether you express it. The real trick is to honestly reframe the situation. There is an ancient story of acceptance that talks about an old man who can no longer work and is dependent on his only son to manage the farm so the family can live. One day, there is an accident and the son breaks both his legs. The villagers weep for the old man and his son – it will be a rough winter if they can't reap the autumn harvest. The old man only smiles and assures everyone that all will be fine. That fall, the emperor calls for every family in the land to send one son to war. Because the old farmer's son is crippled, he cannot go to war, but stays on the farm with his father. The war turns into a massacre. Every son from every village is killed. Except the farmer's son, whose broken legs turned out to be good fortune for the family.

The lesson is that there is no way to predict what will happen down the road. Reacting with anger or stress doesn't help change the future, but letting go of those negative emotions will help keep you healthy. Whenever you find yourself in a situation where you would typically become angry or stressed, notice your reactions. Try to observe yourself objectively and look for a way to respond differently, more positively. Reframe the problem in such a way that you can see the good. For example, you may be sitting in traffic, but at least you aren't the one who was in the car accident that caused the backup . . . accept the boss's reprimand as a chance to improve your performance in the future . . . think of the visit from the in-laws as a chance to let someone else take over the cooking for a night or two . . . realise that the sewer spray was your welcome into a new neighbourhood. That kind of thing.

Another way to reframe the situation is to put little stresses into perspective. After the World Trade Center disaster in September 2001, people reported feeling generally traumatised and worried about personal safety, but they also became 'nicer' on a day-to-day basis. Studies reported that people became more altruistic as their life view changed. Similar things happen when close family members become ill or die – suddenly, the 'little things' that used to bother us fade into the background. It is possible to adopt that kind of attitude even without a major traumatic event to show us what is really important in life. If you find that kind of transition difficult, and you recognise that you tend to become easily angered or stressed, you might want to talk with a psychologist or other professional who can take your individual needs and situation into account and guide you to a healthier way of reacting.

Overeating in Response to Stress:
The Body Shape Connection

Reframing is going to take a lot of practice, especially if you are used to reacting emotionally. While you are working on it, the next best thing you can do is to try to curb your impulse to eat in reaction to stress. Many women eat sweet foods in response to stress. Partly it is a learned habit – many of our mothers gave us cookies or other treats in an attempt to soothe us when we were children, and it usually worked. Even though we've grown up, we still associate those kinds of foods with nurturing and love. Partly, however, eating cookies, candy, ice cream, cakes and similar foods is an attempt to regulate our body chemistry. We are, quite literally, self-medicating with food. Carbohydrates create more 'feel good' brain chemicals, such as serotonin. On a subconscious level, your body knows this, which is why, in times of stress, many of us automatically reach for carbohydrates. We may think that it is because they taste good, but our inner pharmacist is simply trying to find a potion that will knock down our stress reactions.

Eating carbohydrates may be an attempt
to regulate body chemistry.

Interestingly, apple-shaped women may be more prone to this type of stress eating than pear-shaped women. Studies have shown that women who are highly reactive to stress – those who have worse moods and higher levels of cortisol – typically eat more in response to stress. And the foods they eat tend to be sweet. So these high-reacting women (who, we know from previous studies, are probably apple-shaped) eat more in times of stress. The problem is that eating sweet foods when cortisol levels are high is like pouring sugar on top of a chocolate bar – your body is already primed for high blood glucose and high insulin levels due to the cortisol, so eating a sweet food just aggravates your blood glucose levels even more. Insulin levels rise even higher, and you are primed for visceral fat. We know that people who are depressed or under stress for a long time tend to gain weight, in part because of these cortisol, blood glucose and insulin fluctuations.

So it seems that apple-shaped women react more strongly to depression and stress – both physically and emotionally – and that these reactions make them more likely to seek out 'comfort foods' when they are feeling especially vulnerable. And unfortunately, their unique biology already puts them at a health disadvantage. For apple-shaped women, then, eating half a litre of ice cream after a stressful day is exactly the wrong activity. It will *feel* like the right choice, as your inner pharmacist calls for more carbohydrates, but in reality it will only fuel the fire. Already high levels of blood glucose will shoot up higher, already high levels of insulin will climb higher, and their bodies become fat-making machines. You couldn't ask for a more efficient way to build a bigger waist. A better choice for dealing with stress would be to fight the urge for comfort foods and instead go for a long walk, run or cycle to 'eat up' the extra glucose and balance the circulating stress hormones. Then, eat a full, apple-appropriate meal (see chapter 11).

Medications

Another link in the chain that you can tackle is the HPA axis reactivity. Research has shown that the regulatory centres of the HPA axis are affected by smoking, excessive alcohol and depression. Obviously, then, don't smoke, and don't drink more than one or two glasses of any alcoholic beverage per day. If you feel depressed, talk with your physician about whether an antidepressant medication might be right for you. In depression, the neurons of the brain don't communicate properly because not enough neurotransmitters are available to spark the electrical signals. The main depression-related neurotransmitters are serotonin, norepinephrine and dopamine. Together, they regulate mood, pain perception and emotional control. Antidepressant medications work by increasing the availability of one, two or all three of these neurotransmitters at the nerve endings.

Studies have shown that some antidepressants help improve the regulation of the HPA axis. The ones that have been especially effective for this purpose are the tricyclic antidepressants, such as amitriptyline (Elavil) and citalopram (Cipramil). These medications work directly to improve depression, but they also stabilise the reactivity that causes high cortisol levels. In addition, research has shown that some medications may increase metabolism, control appetite and aid in weight loss. For example, the medication Reductil (sibutramine) was originally investigated as an antidepressant, but it proved to be such a valuable tool for the loss of visceral fat that it is currently approved for use as a weight loss medication. Another antidepressant, bupropion, affects norepinephrine and dopamine neurotransmitters. It seems to curb cravings so well that it is used as a stop-smoking aid (under the brand name Zyban), and many women lose weight while taking it. Other antidepressants, such as Prozac (fluoxetine), may not have as strong an effect on the cortisol connection and may actually cause weight gain. One study found that people taking fluoxetine lost weight, but mainly from subcutaneous fat loss – there was very little loss of visceral fat.

Antidepressants that impact both serotonin and norepinephrine neurotransmitters, such as Efexor (venlafaxine) and Cymbalta (duloxetine) – also seem to play a role in relieving the physical symptoms so commonly associated with depression. These include headache, back pain, irritable bowel symptoms, fatigue and many, many other problems that keep us from fully enjoying life. Remember, the pain from these diseases is real. Antidepressants work because they affect the physical body at the level of the neuron or by influencing the HPA axis.

Stress Reduction

Another way to influence the HPA axis is through what scientists call 'mindfulness-based stress reduction'. Researchers tested this relaxation programme on patients with cancer, a population that typically experiences a lot of stress. The participants were taught meditation and yoga and were encouraged to practise these relaxation techniques at home. Before and after the eight-week intervention, researchers measured the participants' cortisol levels, sleep qualit and symptoms of stress. They found that stress symptoms decreased, sleep improved and the pattern of cortisol secretion changed, suggesting that the relaxation programme had some effect on HPA axis activity. Other studies have found that relaxation helps reduce both stress and cortisol levels, regardless of the method. For example, one study found that playing music during a stressful medical procedure helped patients relax, with corresponding lower blood pressure and cortisol levels. Massage, progressive muscle relaxation, tai chi, reading, brisk walking and even watching a humorous video have all been shown to reduce cortisol levels in stressed individuals.

What this says to me is that relaxation – just like stress – is what we make of it. It doesn't matter how you relax, as long as you take time to do something that takes your mind off the stressful events of the day and allows your body time to recover from all its physiologic gymnastics. My guess is that a quiet bubble bath would work equally as well for women who enjoy a warm soak. After looking at the literature, it seems that you need a minimum of 20 minutes of doing whatever it is that relaxes you to reap the positive effects. An hour is even better (unless you're in the bath, and then you'll prune). The critical point is that you need to pay attention to your stress and then do something to reduce its physical effects. Too much stress means high cortisol, which means extra visceral fat. So really, taking a half hour to meditate, read a novel, listen to your favourite music, get a massage, do yoga or enjoy a nature walk is important for waistline control. Consider it as vital to your health as exercise.

Action Items for Chapter 9:
Stress, Anger and Depression

◆ Keep a journal to record your positive and negative emotions and to record stressful experiences. Writing can be a tool for identifying ongoing problems in your life and clarifying exactly what in your life is creating emotional turmoil. Once you understand where your trigger points are, you can take steps to change the situation or change your reactions to them. A study of patients with rheumatoid arthritis found that those who kept a journal felt less pain and functioned better than those who did not write.

◆ Expand your social network. That's the psychological way of saying go out and make some friends. Having a friend to talk things over with is immensely important. Women with good social support networks stay healthier, experience less stress and deal with illnesses better than women who feel isolated. Find people you can trust, people who will really listen when you need to blow off steam or consult about a problem. Ironically, women's number-one complaint against doctors is that they don't listen. We need friends to keep us healthy.

◆ Don't be afraid to seek professional help for problems with anger, stress or depression. There are many different forums for dealing with these problems, including medication (in the case of depression), individual or group therapy, and anger management or stress reduction classes. Because of the health consequences of these emotions, talk with your GP about your concerns and discuss what options might be best for you. Teamwork works best for managing depression – you need to encourage the involvement of a friend or health partner, family members, your GP and a therapist.

◆ If you have diabetes, heart disease or other chronic disease, you should know that stress, anger and depression can exacerbate your symptoms. Blood glucose levels can fluctuate wildly under stressful conditions, and you may find it difficult to keep control. Autoimmune diseases, such as multiple sclerosis, lupus or rheumatoid arthritis, can flare up during times of stress. It is vitally important that you adopt a relaxation method and use it as often as necessary.

◆ Evaluate each new potentially stressful situation. Ask yourself what aspects of the situation are in your control, and which are not. Let go of fretting about things you can't control. Work on fixing what you can control. Not only will you be helping to solve the problem, but you will feel less helpless and frustrated. Depending on your situation, this may mean changing jobs or even careers, going back to school, or resolving to lose 5cm (2in) from your waist. Change can be frightening and difficult, but most people find that the end result is worth the extra effort.

◆ Fight denial. Denial is a powerful state of mind, a critical feature that prevents us from taking positive action. Evaluate your emotional state honestly. If you feel stressed or depressed, talk with friends and family members about it. Recognise that a problem might exist. Then, seek help. The sooner you do, the sooner you'll feel better. And remember, stress, anger and depression affect more than just your state of mind – they help create heart disease and type 2 diabetes, which can shorten your life.

Take to Heart …

◆ Some scientists suggest that part of the reason we are in the middle of an epidemic of obesity is our stressful lives and the cortisol-visceral fat connection. If this is true, then every time we choose to react badly to stressful situations, we are making ourselves fatter. Which means that we may be able to avoid some weight gain simply by shrugging off some of those petty annoyances that used to make us crazy. Can you think of a better reason to try to adopt a more relaxed attitude?

◆ And maybe, with the world so full of uncertainty and bad things, maybe we need to ease up on ourselves a bit. That the world is getting fatter is somewhat understandable, given the current state of affairs. We live in very stressful times, and much of it we can't control. Every day we are bombarded by headlines about bio-terrorism, weapons of mass destruction, kidnappings and murder. Jobs are lost, the economy is slow, and companies are cutting back on retirement benefits. Try as we may, the stress of living gives us all somewhat of an excuse – to be a little fatter than we'd like, perhaps a little angrier, a little more stressed, a little more depressed. If we acknowledge that and understand that we can't control the big things, then it becomes easier just to do our small part on this planet. Find your own way to ease the tension, for yourself and for others. Let someone cut in front of you in a line of traffic . . . give the shop assistant a smile . . . be slower to anger, quicker to forgive. If you are overweight, remember that no one is asking you to become model-thin. Just do your small part to lose a few centi-metres. I want the information in this book to make you healthier and happier, not more neurotic about your weight. Life is hard enough – take a little time to find the things you love to do and then enjoy them. That is the ultimate key to good health.

PART THREE

SOLUTIONS

CHAPTER 10

Eating Well

I was at a garden party last summer when the hostess pulled me aside. When we were alone, she confided that she was finally serious about wanting to get her act together and get healthier. She felt as though she had spent her life caring for other people, and now was the time to take care of herself for a change. 'I know that starts with diet,' she said. 'I just don't know how to start or what to eat. I've read *everything*, but I'm still so confused.' I stared at her in disbelief, and in that moment I realised exactly how inadequate and negligent the media messages about diet have been. This is a vibrant, intelligent, inquisitive woman who has a Ph.D. in psychology. She teaches at a university and counsels others on how to clarify their emotions so that they can take positive steps in their lives. If she was confused about diet and weight loss, then everyone else didn't stand a chance.

It has been my experience that most women are confused about nutrition – not because they have too little information, but because there is just too much to keep straight. Many women feel as though their heads are being whipped around by conflicting reports, leaving them bewildered, frustrated and defeated. 'Why bother changing what I eat because of what I read in the newspaper today?' one woman asked. 'They're just going to tell me something different tomorrow.'

FOOD INFORMATION REALITY CHECK

We are bombarded with health messages every day. Radio, television, internet, magazine and newspapers all give us the 'latest and greatest' food and diet news. One of the unintended side effects is that we can easily become overwhelmed. For example, let's say you resolve to eat more vegetables, and you buy a package of carrots in the grocery store. Well, if you read enough magazines and news articles, you'll discover that different experts will tell you to: (1) wash the carrots instead of peeling them to retain more nutrients; (2) no, peel the carrots instead of washing them to get rid of any dirt and contaminants; (3) steam the carrots instead of boiling them to retain the nutrients; (4) no, boil the carrots, but then use the cooking water to make rice, so that the nutrients from the carrots are absorbed by the grains; (5) no, microwave the carrots in a little water – the shorter cooking time will cut down on nutrient loss; (6) eat only organic carrots to avoid pesticides; (7) cut the carrots crosswise, straight down, instead of diagonally or lengthwise, to minimise the surface area exposed to air, which causes nutrients to be lost due to oxidation; (8) don't eat carrots at all because they have a high glycaemic index. No wonder good health starts feeling like a chore. And no wonder many of us give up trying to understand nutrition.

Ironically, most women are confused about nutrition – not because they have too little information, but because there is just too much to keep straight.

Healthy eating doesn't have to be that difficult. Good health shouldn't require an advanced degree in mathematics to figure out calorie or carb count, glycaemic index, percentage of fat or micrograms of magnesium. When you become obsessed with counting and measuring and numbers, then mealtimes are no longer enjoyable. Food becomes part of the stress of daily life. That's one of the reasons most diets fail in the long run – it is difficult to maintain a high level of interest and commitment if the diet is too intrusive. That's why I don't like talking about numbers, and you'll notice that I do so minimally here. That doesn't mean I won't ask you to change the way you eat; I just won't do it in terms of grams and ounces, or – even worse – percentage of fat, carbs or protein. We can be logical about this, understand food basics and then make healthy changes step by step. Weight loss and good nutrition should be a part of your life; they shouldn't dictate the terms of your life. There's no reason to make yourself neurotic on the way to a healthier you.

Healthy eating doesn't have to be that difficult. Good health shouldn't require an advanced degree in mathematics to count carbs.

If you are an overweight apple-shaped woman, or if you have a waist circumference larger than 90cm (35½in), then you now know that reducing your waist is key to preventing or controlling the metabolic syndrome, type 2 diabetes, cardiovascular disease and maybe even breast and endometrial cancers. If you are an overweight pear-shaped woman, you are probably reassured that a little extra weight isn't as harmful for you as it is for an apple-shaped woman, but you may be interested in losing girth for the sake of appearance or quality of life or to avoid becoming apple-shaped. I can help you with those issues, but only if you are willing to look at weight loss – or better yet, health by the centimetres – from a new perspective.

Perhaps the biggest problem I have with the media's coverage of diet and nutrition information is that the emphasis is always more on short-term weight loss success. We are not taught about long-term investment in our health future. Rather, we are encouraged to think in terms of *quick* – which diet will get you to lose the most weight the fastest. Fifteen kilos by summer? Sure, it can be done. But I would also bet that most of the weight will be back on by New Year's Eve. The human body is not designed to give up weight easily – its survival mechanism wants to retain as much weight as it can. We have to work with our bodies – and the unique physiology that comes from natural body shape – to find realistic solutions to the problems of too much fat.

The human body is not designed to give up weight
easily – its survival mechanism wants to retain as much
weight as it can.

As I've been saying throughout this book, apple- and pear-shaped women have different needs. Let's start fresh here.

A one-size-fits-all, cookie-cutter diet may be simple, but
it's silly. I don't prescribe medications or hormones
with a one-size-fits-all approach, so why would I
recommend a diet that way?

The nutrition information, tips and eating plans that follow here and in the next two chapters are designed to:

1. help all women get out of the cycle of diet failure;
2. help apple-shaped women reduce their waist size, lower their

risk of getting heart disease and type 2 diabetes, and dampen stress-related eating and weight gain;

3. help pear-shaped women avoid becoming apple-shaped while reducing their risk of osteoporosis;

4. help all women reduce their risk of geting cancer, frailty and other nutrition-related disorders; and

5. give all women the tools they need to make conscious, informed, healthy choices about food *while still living in the real world*. No more fads. No more confusion.

Ready?

NUTRITION BASICS: START FROM THE BEGINNING

There are a few basic principles that underlie all weight loss efforts. If you understand these, everything becomes much clearer.

Peel back all the confusing layers of information about food and weight loss, and at the centre you'll see the *calorie*. Forget everything else for a moment – forget fats and carbs, forget vitamins and minerals, forget fruits and vegetables. I'll get to those later. Let's concentrate on the calorie.

A calorie is simply a unit of energy-producing potential – when you 'burn' a calorie, you release that energy. It works similarly to petrol in a car – the petrol is the fuel, full of energy-producing potential. When you turn on the engine and burn the petrol, the energy is released and the car runs. We all need a certain number of calories, or energy potential, every day just to carry on the duties of living – breathing, swallowing, sitting, walking, blinking, et cetera. Every minute we are alive we are burning calories, and the more we do, the more calories we burn. We burn calories while we are sleeping, but we burn more when we are awake. We burn calories while we are sitting down, but more while we are standing. In a nutshell, the more you demand of your muscles, the more calories you burn. If you decide to run a marathon, you'll need a tremendous number of calories just to make it through the race.

We get calories from food. So at the most fundamental level, the purpose of food is to supply us with enough energy (in the form of calories) to live. Ideally, we strive for balance. Getting too few calories means that we won't be giving our bodies enough energy to function properly – our metaphorical cars run out of petrol. Eating too many calories leads to the problem of what to do with the excess. A car has a limited storage capacity for petrol. If you try to overfill it, the gas will spill out onto the ground. But our bodies have an unlimited storage capacity – we simply turn the excess calories into fat. The fat can be turned back into energy any time it is needed. In countries where the food supply is unreliable, this ability to store up fat allows us to feast and fatten up in times of plenty, and then draw on the fat energy reserves to survive in times of famine.

Most of us never face famine. Food is abundant, and we eat every day. Most of us would panic if we were forced to miss two meals in a row. But our bodies still function on the same principle – store fat in case of emergency. So if we eat too many calories, we put on fat. It doesn't matter whether those calories come from hamburgers, bagels, chocolate bars, cheese or tofu. Too many calories lead to excess fat.

Why Counting Calories Is Difficult

Which leads to the next obvious question: How many calories are 'too many'? Cumulative data tell us that the average woman requires about 2,000 calories per day to live. That is, if an average woman ate 2,000 calories' worth of food per day, she would not gain weight, nor would she lose weight. She would be in perfect balance, with her daily activities burning up exactly the same number of calories she took in.

If she ate less than 2,000 calories per day, she would lose weight; and if she ate more than 2,000 calories per day, she would gain weight. The equation really is that simple. If you eat more food calories than you burn, you will gain weight. Apple-shaped women will be more likely to gain weight as visceral fat around their waists, and pear-shaped women will be more likely to gain subcutaneous fat around their lower bodies. Conversely, if you burn more calories than you eat, you will lose weight. That is the whole secret to weight loss. But – and you knew there would be a 'but' – the reality of that kind of calorie balance is very difficult, for several reasons.

First, the precise number of calories you burn changes from day to day depending on what you are doing. If you spend a day lounging at the beach, you'll burn fewer calories than you would on an average day working in an office or running errands at home. On the other hand, if you spend the day swimming and playing at the beach, you'll likely burn more calories than you would on an average day. Because we don't have an internal counter that tells us exactly how many calories we are burning, we have to estimate how much to eat, and we don't do that very well.

Second, knowing the exact calorie count of everything you eat is nearly impossible. Remember, calories are in all foods. So if you want to know the precise number of calories in that hamburger you ate for lunch, you'll have to know how big the hamburger was in grams, then what kind of bun it was on, and don't forget to include the calories in ketchup, mayonnaise, relish, cheese or any other toppings. Then add in any calories from your drink, assuming you know how many milli-litres you drank, and any side dishes. If you ate French fries, how many did you eat? How large were they – thin cut, thick or shoestring? All those factors contribute to calorie count. Keeping track of all your daily calories is a Herculean task. Women who have done it – for example, women who have recovered from anorexia nervosa, the psychological disorder that causes them to eat so little that they drop to dangerously low body weights – describe the amount of time and effort it took for them to monitor calories as *exhausting*. It is not worth spending that much of your life tallying numbers.

The third reason why calorie balance is difficult is that every person is unique. It's important for scientists to know that an average woman burns 2,000 calories per day, but who is average? How many calories do you burn every day? I'm sure you've known women who eat lunches big enough to feed a rugby player without gaining weight. And there are others who seem to get fatter while eating the same amount as everyone else, the ones who joke that they 'gain five pounds just by smelling a piece of chocolate cake'. The difference is *metabolism*. The official definition of metabolism is that it is the sum total of all the chemical processes going on in the body. The more casual definition is that metabolism is the rate at which you burn off calories – someone with a 'fast' metabolism burns more calories in an average day than someone with a 'slow' metabolism.

METABOLISM: THE FIRE INSIDE

Metabolism is set, in part, by our genetics, so we each have a general tendency towards having a fast, slow or average metabolism. But part of the burn rate of our metabolism is variable, determined by the chemical processes occurring in the body. These chemical reactions happen every time you move or think – your brain alone requires about 500 calories per day just to keep working. The more you move, the more chemical reactions occur, so your metabolism will temporarily speed up. But if you want to generally keep your metabolism revving higher, you'll need to change your body composition.

Body composition refers to the relative proportion of muscle (called *lean body tissue* or *lean body mass*) and fat. The more lean body tissue we have, the faster our metabolism will be. As discussed in previous chapters, we naturally lose lean muscle mass as we get older, which is one of the reasons we tend to gain weight as we age. We eat the same amount we always have, but our lean body mass has decreased, so we don't burn as many calories as we used to. One way to increase your metabolism is to increase your lean body mass, which requires regular moderate exercise.

If you want to generally keep your metabolism revving higher, you'll need to change your body composition — more muscle and less fat.

Another way to increase your metabolism is to keep the same amount of lean body tissue, but lose fat so that you have proportionately more muscle than fat. Most of us try to do this by drastic dieting, and we do lose fat . . . for the short term, anyway. The medical data are fuzzy about what really happens to metabolism after dieting, but the consensus seems to be that metabolism decreases for two reasons. First, we lose lean body mass. When you go on a low-calorie diet, your body burns fat. But while you are shedding fat, the body also starts to break down muscle tissue so you are also losing lean body mass – and less lean body mass equals lower metabolism. Taken to the extreme, women with anorexia can lose so much muscle tissue that eventually they start to break down heart tissue, and they can die of heart failure. This same kind of self-cannibalism happens with any very low-calorie diet – we break down our own muscles for nutrients.

The second reason metabolism slows down has to do with the famine effect – a biological drive for survival. Remember, the whole reason the body stores extra calories as fat is to protect us in times of famine. Losing weight might make us happy, but our bodies start to worry that there really is a famine. Why else would your fat stores be dropping so quickly or so low? According to the physiologic laws of survival, weight loss is bad because if the 'famine' continues, the skinniest people will die first. Therefore, the body does what it must to preserve energy. For some people, it may mean an increase in the cues for hunger, which the body hopes will drive us to eat. (And, very often, we do, which is why some people go off their diets and binge once in a while.) For other people, it may mean that metabolism slows down so that the body conserves energy. People who go on very low-calorie diets – less than 1,000 calories per day – are basically putting the brakes on metabolism. As far as the body is concerned, starvation is imminent, so it lowers the number of calories it burns per day. The result is that our bodies work against us to preserve fat, and our weight loss reaches a plateau. Those infamous 'last 10 pounds' won't come off. Still, we're happy to have lost at least some weight, and eventually we go off the diet.

WHY THE WEIGHT COMES BACK

So now you are thinner than you were, and you start to eat your regular diet. Normal food, normal amounts. But remember, your metabolism has slowed down to prepare for long-term famine. Guess what happens. The calories pile up because you aren't burning them as fast. Plus, your body starts to recognise that the famine is over, so hunger soars. You never knew how hungry you were until you gave up dieting. Within a few months, you probably will have regained all the weight you lost, and because your metabolism was temporarily slowed you may gain even more. This is part of the reason why 85 per cent of all people who lose weight regain every kilo within a couple of years.

This metabolism depression can last a very long time. Weight will continue to creep up on you. So you go on another diet . . . lose weight . . . slow your metabolism . . . go off the diet . . . regain even more weight . . . go back on a diet . . . and on and on. No one should have to go through that agony again and again. It's like a version of Hell – think Sisyphus, the tragic figure of Greek mythology condemned for eternity to roll a boulder up a mountain only to have it roll back down to the bottom so he has to start pushing all over again. How many diet boulders have you pushed in your lifetime?

Many experts recommend exercising while you diet to avoid that metabolic slowdown. I'll also recommend exercise, but for more than just that one reason. Actually, the research on what happens when you mix exercise and diet has given perplexing results. It is logical to think that if you go on a low-calorie diet (which lowers metabolism) and also start exercising (which raises metabolism by preserving muscle mass), the two would balance out to keep metabolism at an even keel. The reality is a little more complicated than that. Some research has demonstrated that exercise plus a *moderate* diet may help counterbalance the loss of lean body mass. That's because the human body requires a certain amount of food *in addition to* exercise to conserve the high-revving lean body mass while losing fat. But if you don't eat enough, all the exercise in the world won't help your metabolism stay high.

Taking off weight doesn't have to be torture – you just have to know the tricks.

So here's your good news for the day: very low-calorie dieting is not your best choice for lasting weight loss. You may take off weight very quickly, but you'll also regain it in short order. It's like when a person has the flu or a stomach virus that doesn't allow her to eat for several days. The 'flu diet' has been known to help women lose two, three or even four kilos in a single week, and yet all that weight is back within another week or two. It's just the way we are built. Taking off weight doesn't have to be torture – you just have to know the tricks.

MIND OVER MUFFINS

Yes, there are tricks. This whole need-to-burn-more-calories-than-we-eat fact is not new. I'm sure you've heard it before, even if you never fully understand all the nuances. And yet, 75 per cent of all Britons are overweight (with a BMI of 25 or more). The problem certainly isn't lack of knowledge. Walk into any hospital or surgery and observe the number of overweight physicians and nurses; you'll find quite a few. These are people who make their living dispensing health advice. If the equation is so simple, why aren't we all thin?

Our society is not designed to keep you healthy ...
there are few supports for people who truly want to
pursue wellness.

Part of the reason is that, as we all intuitively know, there is more to eating than just knowing about calories. Food plays a central role in our lives – it is part of every celebration and ceremony, it can express our ethnic heritage and traditions and it brings families together. We give gifts of food to express love or friendship. Cooking can be a point of pride, a creative outlet, or even part of a healing ritual – the medicinal power of chicken soup comes from its preparation as much as its ingredients. Food and weight are societal problems as much as individual ones.

It is a sad fact that our society is not designed to keep you healthy. Sure, we have wonderful physicians and other health care workers who will try to cure you when you are sick, but there are few supports for people who want to pursue wellness. Real world nutrition guidance is especially lacking. When was the last time you saw a television commercial for a healthy food? There have been a few – ads for milk, orange juice and porridge come to mind – but they are rare. What we have is a nearly steady stream of media messages designed to encourage you to buy foods that are unhealthy.

Food Myths

If you don't have a basic understanding of the forces working to try to control your eating, you don't stand a chance in this world. Messages that are among the most dangerous try to trick or seduce you into eating foods that are high in calories, foods that are more likely to cause weight gain. These messages include:

◆ **Fun.** Ideally, food is flavourful, nutritious, filling, satisfying and memorable. It can't really be 'fun'. Watch television commercials that tell you a particular food is fun, and you're likely to see people dancing or laughing hysterically while they eat. You'll see them tossing the food in the air, or the food itself transforms into a cartoon object. The food will draw crowds, create instant parties and make the eater popular. In reality, we know that no food can make us dance or laugh, but the images are so powerful. They make us wish our lives were that carefree and happy. Even if we don't consciously remember the dancing and laughing, the general good feelings evoked by the commercials will carry over into the supermarket. We pick the product up off the shelf, somehow feel good about our decision, and bring it home. It's as though someone were casting a happy spell on us whenever we look at the product. Once you become aware of the 'fun' messages, the subconscious spell is broken.

◆ **Reward.** Using food as a reward is a sure way to become overweight. There's no doubt about it – food is enjoyable. That's what makes it *work* as a reward. We learned this when we were young when our parents rewarded us with our favourite foods if we behaved. But when we use food as a tool instead of as a way of nourishing our bodies, then it becomes an object of desire, something positive to attain. But instead of winning a blue ribbon for our efforts, we win an extra few centimetres of fat on our thighs or waist. It is OK to splurge on a high-calorie food once in a while, but it's important to be conscious of when and why you are doing it. You never 'deserve' a piece of cake. You don't have to win it or earn it. Food should never be a prize. Eat it, or don't eat it, but don't rationalise it. Be wary of products that seduce you with a message of how deserving you are – they are playing with your emotions, trying to make you feel deprived even when you might otherwise be perfectly content.

It is OK to splurge on a high-calorie food once in a while, but it's important to be conscious of when and why you are doing it.

◆ **Energy.** All foods contain energy because all foods contain calories. Remember, a calorie is simply a unit of energy-producing potential – when you 'burn' a calorie, you release that energy. There are many, many advertisements for foods that purport to 'give you energy'. In reality, no food can give you energy beyond what you get from calories – not vitamins, not minerals, not herbs, not caffeine. If a product is said to give energy, it must be high in calories. That's why it is legal (and honest) for a chocolate bar to claim to give you energy. It doesn't mean that it is necessarily healthy for you, just that it has a lot of calories – usually in the form of sugar.

◆ **Beauty.** It always amazes me to see toothpick-thin young women on television shows or advertisements casually eating half a litre of ice cream or large helpings of pizza. We know in our heads that these are just images, and that the actresses weren't really eating all that food – it was acting. When the camera stopped rolling, they spat out whatever was in their mouths. No one can eat as much of the kinds of treat foods we see being eaten on television and still be that thin. This sets up an unobtainable standard of beauty – a size-8 life full of indulgences. In reality, it is impossible. We cannot eat incessantly and unthinkingly without gaining weight. We know that, and yet we are fooled again and again. In the 1990s, when the tobacco companies came under fire for using advertisements to entice children into starting to smoke, they adopted a voluntary marketing code. One of the outcomes was that in the United States one rarely sees healthy, active people smoking in ads any more. (In Britain *all* smoking ads in all media have been banned since 2003.) No more water-skiing smokers, football-playing smokers or anything else that would suggest that smokers get some active health benefit from cigarettes. I'd like to see the same type of code enacted for eating – no more skinny models eating potato crisps in an aggressive frenzy, no more weightless angels popping cakes into their mouths. Truth in advertising has to extend to food.

◆ **Bigger.** When did we ever lose sight of the wise adage *less is more*? Now, everything is supersized. It seems like a good deal for you, but did you ever wonder why the fast-food companies bother to give you so much more food for so little money? Trust me, it's not for your benefit. It has to be worth money to those companies, otherwise the practice wouldn't continue. They make incremental pence on that single supersize purchase, but their main goal is to build an army of loyal customers who will return again and again. How do you build a better customer for fast food? Simple. Make her fat so that she needs to eat more. (It's just like building a customer for cigarettes – entice young women with images of glamour or the empty promise of weight loss and then continue to sell cigarettes long after they are addicted.) With inexpensive food so easily available, it becomes a cheap and easy meal solution to pop into the local burger outlet for enough food to satisfy. We've been marketed into the next-size jeans. And in case you didn't notice, part of the allure of fast-food restaurants is the promise of 'fun'.

Food Psychology

Another place that the bigger-is-better motif has gone crazy is in the American warehouse buying clubs, and the cash and carry stores patronised by employees of some British companies. Don't get me wrong – I'm all for saving money on 64 rolls of toilet paper or that gallon jar of mustard – but unhealthy food in big packages is bad news. One behavioural study investigated the differences in how much and how fast people used up their purchases of juice or cookies. Some shoppers bought regular-sized packages, but other shoppers bought the large, convenience-sized packages. Results showed that the average daily consumption of juice and cookies approximately *doubled* when shoppers bought the large promotional packages. Not only did they eat more per sitting, but *they ate the food more often.* The same was true for buying two-for-one promotional items. They are no deal for our waistlines because we don't buy them half as often – we just eat them twice as fast. This is only true for products that are easy to eat, such as crisps, biscuits, pretzels, chocolate bars, and other snack foods. Buying and freezing large quantities of chicken breasts doesn't change how often people eat chicken.

Out of Sight, Out of Mind

Additional research showed that people tend to eat even *more* if the food is visible. Here's a setup that will probably sound familiar to some people. Researchers tested how many chocolate 'kisses' [a type of small American sweet] were eaten during the course of a week under three different conditions: (1) the jar of sweets was placed on each participant's desk so it was visible and within reach; (2) the jar of sweets was placed in the participant's desk drawer so that it was not visible, but it was still within reach; and (3) the jar of chocolates was placed on a shelf about 2m (6ft) away so that it was visible, but not within reach. As you might expect, people with chocolate on top of their desks ate about

50 per cent more than those who kept the candy in a drawer, but they ate nearly *three times as much chocolate* as the people who had the candy far away on a shelf. This means that large packages of readily available cookies or sweets really do call out to us. They subconsciously draw our attention over and over again. And with large quantities, there is little chance of running out, so we feel freer to indulge.

Say 'When'

Remember that last sentence because it will serve you well as you try to slim: with large quantities, we feel freer to indulge. We like to think that we eat when we are hungry, and we stop when we are satisfied. Unfortunately, that's not exactly true. We eat for a number of different reasons, not just hunger. Some women eat when they are happy, others eat when they are depressed. Many of us eat when we are stressed, both as a way of seeking comfort and as a way of self-medicating ourselves – many common comfort foods boost the production of the feel-good chemical serotonin in the brain. We eat when we are bored or at a party or because it happens to be lunchtime. Sometimes we eat just to enjoy the taste of food, the same way some people go to a museum to take in the visual pleasures of art.

Even the feeling of being satisfied or 'full' doesn't always come naturally. Distractions can prevent us from feeling the internal cues that tell us when we've had enough. For example, studies have shown that people tend to eat more when they sit with other people than when they are alone. We also eat more if there are more choices – such as at an all-you-can-eat buffet, or if the meal has five courses instead of three. And we eat more when more is presented to us, even when we try to let hunger be our guide.

Disconnected from Hunger

Food psychologist Dr Brian Wansink of the University of Illinois at Urbana-Champaign conducted several ingenious studies to demonstrate how much we rely on visual cues, instead of hunger, to stop eating. In one study, he outfitted soup bowls with hidden tubes so that they could be secretly refilled as people ate the soup. Some people in the study ate from a refillable bowl, others ate from a regular bowl, but all were instructed to eat as much as they wanted. People who ate from the never-ending bowl of soup ate *40 per cent more* on average than people who ate from regular bowls. They seemed to judge when to stop by the level of the soup in the bowl, instead of the quantity of soup in their stomachs.

In a different study, people who went to see a movie were given a coupon for free popcorn and a fizzy drink when they purchased their ticket. At the snack stand, the unwitting participants received either a medium-sized or a large-sized container of popcorn. At the end of the movie, the containers were collected to measure how much popcorn had been eaten. In addition, each participant was asked to complete a questionnaire about how much they liked the taste of the popcorn. Those who received the large-sized container of popcorn ate about 50 per cent more popcorn than those who received the medium-sized container – *even when they reported that they hadn't liked the taste*. In fact, the study was repeated with some moviegoers receiving stale, two-week-old popcorn, and they still ended up eating more of it when they received large-sized containers. That's how powerful external cues are in their ability to blur our perceptions of hunger. Bigger packages make us eat more, just as unendingly large bowls of soup make us eat more. The lesson is that we are not very good at judging our hunger level. I believe that part of our collective weight problem may come from all the distractions we have in our lives, and from the extra-big portions of food currently available.

Supersized Servings

Studies confirm that portions in American restaurants and in serving sizes of packaged goods have gone up considerably in recent years. A study published in a 2003 issue of the *Journal of the American Dietetic Association* compared today's average serving sizes of fast foods, packaged foods and bread products with the standard serving sizes recommended by the U.S. Food and Drug Administration (FDA). Get this – the average serving of French fries is twice as big as the FDA-recommended servings, an average bagel is about three times as big as the FDA-sized bagel and the average chocolate chip cookie is about four times as big.

Other U.S. researchers compared today's standard serving sizes to those in the 1970s. They looked at the sizes of portions served at home or in fast-food and family-style restaurants. They discovered that portion sizes have increased for all foods checked except pizza – the size of a standard pizza decreased slightly. For all other foods, portion sizes got significantly bigger. On average, present-day portions load Americans up with about 35 per cent more calories than was eaten in 1977. For example, a standard portion of salty snacks (such as potato crisps or corn chips) increased in size by a whopping 60 per cent. For this one product alone, we are eating 93 more calories per serving than we did in 1977.

Portions in Britain are generally smaller than those in the United States, although some packaged snacks and sweets have increased in size in recent years. Also, the widespread habit of spending hours in front of the television tends to encourage snacking (while, of course, doing nothing to burn up calories). So Britons, like Americans, have been increasing their calorie intake.

Going back to those hypothetical 93 extra calories – what could this change really mean for an individual?

It could mean about 4.5kg (10lb) per year.

Consider this: when the body stores excess calories as fat, it takes about 7,700 excess calories to create a kilo of fat. So if you eat an extra 93 calories per day every day for a year, you will gain roughly 4.5kg

(10lb) at the end of that year (93 calories x 365 days/year = 33,945 extra calories, divide by 7,700 calories/kilo of fat = 4.5kg [10lb] of fat). Just to make this clear, 93 calories is about one shortbread round. Or about nine potato crisps. Or about six French fries. Or two-thirds of a can of fizzy drink. So if you started eating one additional shortbread round each day as a snack, you will gain about 4.4kg (10lb) in a year. On the other hand, if you normally drink a regular can of fizzy drink every day and then stop, you will lose about 6kg (13½lb) in a year – *without dieting or doing anything else.* (One 330ml [11½fl oz] can of cola = 130 calories x 365 = 47,450 calories, divide by 7,700 calories/kilo of fat = 6kg (13½lb) of fat.)

This means that all those increased portion sizes add up over time. If you're wondering how those extra 10, 15 or more kilos sneaked up on you, it may have been partly due to larger portion sizes. And remember – with large quantities, we feel freer to indulge. So we get served bigger portions in restaurants, we make more food at home, we buy snacks in bulk, packages contain more food and many of us don't stop eating until we are finished.

We live in an environment that encourages eating, and chances are that's not going to change anytime soon. But once you are aware of the weight that can result from larger portions, you can fight back with some psychological tactics of your own:

◆ Don't 'supersize'. If you have an option for a larger portion, say no. Don't be tempted by the small incremental price – you'll end up paying much more than that if you have to buy new, larger-sized clothing.

◆ Eat out less often so that you control the portion sizes.

◆ At home, serve yourself and your family, then put the rest of the food away. Your family can always get second helpings if they are still hungry, but everyone will be less likely to reach for more if the food is less visible and less convenient.

◆ Avoid buffet-style restaurants if possible. The large array of foods is an invitation to overeat. And too many of us feel the urge to 'get my money's worth' at all-you-can-eat restaurants, which can override all your nutrition savvy.

◆ If you shop at one of the cash and carry stores, avoid buying snack foods there. Buy the smaller bags or boxes at the regular grocery store. Or, buy the larger-sized bag or box and then repackage the foods into smaller resealable bags or plastic storage boxes when you get home.

◆ Of course, no one really needs to keep cookies, cakes, crisps or other snacks in the house. We buy them by habit or because we think our children 'need' them. My first recommendation is to remove all snacks from the house. But I realise that that isn't an option for many families. So if you have snacks, put them all into a separate cupboard, away from the healthier foods so that you don't see them every time you go to your kitchen. Out of sight really is out of mind.

◆ Put all food on a plate before eating it – that goes for cookies, crisps, pretzels, sweets or any other snack. You are much more likely to overeat if you mindlessly dip into a bag or box.

THE 25 PER CENT SOLUTION

So we are all battling portion sizes, dieting dilemmas and the threat of lower metabolism. Part of the solution is within everyone's reach.

According to the best research, if you want to lose weight and *keep the weight off* without slowing your metabolism, you need to do moderate exercise and restrict calories by *no more than* 25 per cent. That means that by eliminating just one-quarter of everything you already eat, you will be losing weight in a healthier way than if you started measuring out cups of rice or grams of breakfast cereal. Cutting back more will take weight off faster, but you'll just put it back on relatively quickly. I call this the '25 per cent solution', and it is your best bet for breaking out of diet hell.

If you want to lose weight and keep the weight off without slowing your metabolism, you need to do moderate exercise and restrict calories by no more than 25 per cent.

Here's the way the 25 per cent solution works: pretend that you are going to have a normal meal. Put your usual amount of food on your plate, then remove one-quarter of everything. Take off one-quarter of the peas, one-quarter of the mashed potatoes, one-quarter of the pork chop, one-quarter of everything. Do the same thing with dessert. Put all those little one-quarter servings away as leftovers, or throw them away. Don't think of it as throwing away food – think of it as throwing away your fat. If you have soup, either measure out one-quarter of the total amount in a liquid measuring jug or do your best to spoon off what you estimate to be one-quarter of the whole bowl. This doesn't require precision – just estimate the quarter portion. Don't leave it on the table – wrap it up and put it out of sight immediately. It will be too tempting if it is sitting right there in front of you. If you are eating at a restaurant, ask the server to bring a to-go box or bag to the table with the meal and then separate and store one-quarter of your meal before you start eating. Or place it on a separate plate and ask the server to take it away. If you do this at every meal and with every snack you will automatically reduce your calories by 25 per cent.

The only thing you have to remember with this technique is that you can't overload your plate with the intention of eliminating 25 per cent – you have to pretend you are eating a typical meal. You also can't eat any additional snacks, nothing over what you would usually eat. If you now have a bagel or a chocolate bar for a mid-afternoon snack, just cut away one-quarter and eat the rest. But don't start eating a bagel or a chocolate bar if you don't already do so because you'll end up adding more calories than you are cutting away. The goal is to eat with your family without totally giving up the foods you love, while still losing weight. I'll give you guidance about your food choices in the next chapters – for right now, just cut away one-quarter of everything you eat.

If you diligently apply the 25 per cent solution, you can't help but lose girth and inches. The equation is simple: when you reduce the total number of calories you eat each day by a manageable proportion, your body will start dipping into its fat stores for energy, and your waistline will gradually decrease. The 25 per cent solution works slowly, but it works. It allows your body to adjust to a new amount of food without drastically cutting calories. This is the simplest, most fundamental way to lose the centimetres, something anyone can do, even if you have minimal motivation. Ideally, you'll pair this with exercise (see chapter 13) so that you hold on to as much lean body mass as possible.

If you diligently apply the 25 per cent solution, you
can't help but lose weight and girth.

After about three weeks, the smaller portion sizes will look normal to you, and most people find they can't imagine how they ever ate more. The long-term benefit will be lasting weight loss, without having to count calories or starve. In fact, if you find yourself constantly hungry, you're doing something wrong.

BEFORE YOU BEGIN YOUR
BODY SHAPE PROGRAMME

The next two chapters contain the body shape eating programmes for apple- and pear-shaped women. My diet recommendations are based on the most up-to-date nutrition and medical research available. I'll tell you which foods are healthier for you, which foods to avoid, and *why*.

These programmes are less structured than other diet programmes for two main reasons. First, I want you to be able to enjoy your life while still becoming healthier. One of the drawbacks of many diet plans is that they assume an all-or-nothing attitude. Too often, then, we end up choosing 'nothing'. Whatever your current level of weight, health or fitness, doing anything is better than doing nothing. These programmes allow you to choose exactly how much you want to participate, and your results will reflect your commitment.

Second, I'm assuming that you are an adult. You make decisions about what to eat every day, several times each day. Each decision has ramifications for your total health. Whenever possible, I provide options so that you can be as diligent as you want to be, depending on the circumstances of the day.

Both programmes also list foods you should avoid whenever possible. These are foods that will undermine your attempts to lose inches and prevent disease. However, I understand that some of your absolute favourite foods may be on that list, and that it is impossible to avoid all 'treat' foods all the time. Even the most avid healthy eaters have their food weaknesses. How easily you can avoid these foods will depend on how often you eat them now. For example, if you never eat potato crisps then it won't be a strain to avoid them. But if you have a bag of crisps with your lunch every day, then it will be much more of an effort for you.

Nutritionists say that these types of foods should be eaten no more than once every six months. I believe that's rather harsh and probably impossible for most people. My ideal recommendation is that you work up to eating no more than one serving of a single off-limits food once a week. That means on a weekly basis, for example, you'll have to decide whether you'd rather drink a can of fizzy drink *or* eat a doughnut *or* have a bag of potato crisps – one per week. That would be the best action. But if you currently eat a lot of off-limits foods, then you'll have to taper down. If you change your diet too much or too quickly, you'll feel frustrated and deprived, which often leads to breaking the diet.

A good option, then, is to reduce how often you eat these foods. What that means for you depends on your current eating habits. If you eat off-limits foods at every meal, start cutting down by eating them at only one meal. I've known people who have had very good results controlling their weight by allowing themselves to eat anything they want, but only on the weekends. All week long they eat only healthy foods, and on the weekends they give themselves permission to eat whatever they like. Although this sounds like diet suicide, most people don't end up on a food binge. They look forward to the change of pace and enjoy a couple of treat foods once a week. One person I know who used to eat something sweet after every meal vowed to eat desserts only on the weekends. He lost 4.5kg (10lb) within three months without making any other changes in his diet. Once you get used to only eating treat foods on the weekends, cut it down by another day so that you eat treats only on Sunday.

PREPARING FOR CHANGE

There are two preparation phases that are important for a successful diet experience. These are appropriate for both apple-shaped women and pear-shaped women.

Phase 1: Food Awareness

For the first week, I don't want you to do anything different from what you normally do except to *pay attention to food*. Eat what you would typically eat, shop for the same items you usually shop for, but do it with awareness.

◆ **Spy in the supermarket.** Go grocery shopping at least once this week and take a look in everyone else's trolley. Quickly try to categorise shoppers as 'healthy' or 'unhealthy' based on the types of foods they have in their trolleys. If someone were looking in your trolley, how would you be categorised?

◆ **Pay attention to what you are eating.** As you sit down to a meal or a snack, remind yourself of what you are doing. Say out loud, 'I am about to eat a salad, a chicken breast, some mashed potatoes, and peas,' or 'I am about to eat a chocolate bar.' If you take seconds, say it out loud again, 'I am about to have a second helping of mashed potatoes.' This is not to make you feel guilty, but to make you aware of the fact that you are eating and what you are eating. For many people, eating becomes as automatic as breathing. By saying the words out loud before eating, you guarantee that you are thinking about the food. If you are eating someplace where this would not be appropriate, take a moment to say the words silently to yourself.

◆ **Write it all down.** Some dietitians recommend writing in a food journal where you can keep a running log of everything you eat. If this sounds like something you would like to do, please do so. It can be very helpful for people who have a visual style of learning – the journal allows them to see, in words, what their diet looks like. For them, a journal is really nothing more than writing 'out loud' what it is they are eating, allowing them greater focus. Other people find the process too tedious. I know one woman who ate *worse* while she kept a food journal because it was easier to write down 'bag of potato crisps' than to list all the foods in a healthy meal. Remember, part of your goal is to make eating a natural activity again. If writing is helpful to you, do it. If not, don't.

◆ **Recognise hunger.** At every meal and before every snack, before taking your first bite, pause a moment to notice your hunger level. What are the feelings in your body that let you know you are hungry? Is your stomach growling? Do you feel light-headed? Do you feel hungry at all? Many people eat when they are not hungry either because they are bored, or because it is mealtime, or because other people are encouraging them to eat. There are some people who don't even know what real hunger feels like because they've never gone that long between meals. Until you understand what your personal hunger cues are, you will not be able to make informed food decisions. So this week, I just want you to notice what the physical feelings of hunger are for you.

◆ **Take a mid-meal breather.** When you have finished half of your dinner, put down your cutlery, place your hands on your lap and take a moment to re-evaluate your hunger level – just a quick 30-second breather to see how the physical feelings of hunger have changed in the middle of dinner. You don't have to do this at breakfast or lunch. Once a day is plenty. And because most people do their worst overeating after 6 P.M., I want you to start being aware of hunger cues in the evening.

Continue all these individual steps throughout the programme. After a couple of weeks, you will find that you have a new relationship with food.

Phase 2: Emotional Preparation

For the second week, continue to pay attention to food and hunger, but now start to prepare your home and your life for the changes that are about to take place.

◆ **Start to apply the 25 per cent solution.**

◆ **Clean out your larder and cupboards.** Take a look at your family's food supply. Reorganise your kitchen so that the healthy foods are separate from the unhealthy foods. For example, keep biscuits, crisps and other snacks in a separate sweets cupboard.

◆ **Learn to leave something behind on your plate at dinner.** I don't care if you leave behind one bean, a single chip or half your hamburger. Too many of us were brought up to become lifelong members of the Clean Plate Club. We were guilt-tripped into finishing every last bite because there were starving children in Africa or Asia. (For me, it was the starving children in China, and I always wondered how the food we didn't eat would get to them.) As a result, many of us still find it difficult to leave even a scrap of food on the plate. You have to get over that. The ultimate goal is going to be for you to eat until you are no longer hungry, not until your plate is clean. Start small. Leave a kernel of sweetcorn. Just let it sit there. Stare at it. Understand that no one will be better off if you eat it – not you, and certainly not the starving children of the world. Enjoy the sense of power that comes from leaving something behind.

◆ **Plan ahead.** As you read through the food choice recommendations for your body shape, make a shopping list of the new foods you want to incorporate into your diet or substitute for other foods. If you make the list while you are reading, you'll be less likely to forget specific items later. Let your enthusiasm now guide your shopping later.

◆ **Keep the plan in sight.** Make photocopies of the food charts and tape them to the inside of a kitchen cupboard or larder door – someplace where you can refer to them when you need them. Use them to improve your eating habits at a pace that works for you and for your weight-loss and taste needs.

◆ **Stay open to new recipes.** Some of the foods recommended on the list might be new to you, or you might not know how to cook within the recommended guidelines. One of the best-kept recipe secrets on the internet is found at www.epicurious.com. There, you can search through more than 16,000 recipes to find exactly what you are looking for by ingredient or other cooking parameters. For example, if you go to the 'Advanced Search' section, you can find low-fat or meatless recipes that contain the exact ingredients you select. Some of the recipes are complex and involved, but others are basic, simple and fast. It is a wonderful resource for people who are just beginning to explore new foods, or who want to expand their already considerable repertoire.

ALCOHOL AND YOUR HEALTH

If you don't currently drink, don't start. But if you enjoy a glass of wine with your dinner, I have good news. Moderate alcohol consumption – one or two units of alcohol per day – can reduce the risk of heart attack by up to half. It also can improve insulin sensitivity and reduce triglycerides, and it seems to help reduce the risk of type 2 diabetes in premenopausal women. One glass of alcohol a day may also help build bone mass – but be aware that more than two glasses per day is harmful to bones. All-in-all, moderate alcohol consumption can be a potentially valuable health aid for apple- and pear-shaped women.

Although these results extend to all types of alcohol, I only recommend wine – with a particular emphasis on red wine, which has additional phytochemicals that make it even healthier. Hard alcohol is too easy to abuse, and beer can contribute to flatulence in many women.

Because drinking alcohol has been associated with a slightly higher risk of breast cancer, I recommend limiting or avoiding alcohol if you have a strong family history of breast cancer.

Remember, all the good effects happen only with about one glass of wine per day. If you drink more than two glasses of wine daily, the effects reverse, with a higher risk of type 2 diabetes, cardiovascular disease and breast cancer.

THE NEXT STEP

The body shape diets outlined in the next two chapters are meant to be a way of life, not a time-limited plan. I understand that this may require some big changes, but there is no reason to go back to your old style of eating. On these diets, you will never be hungry because there is a class of foods that you can eat in unlimited amounts. And trust me – once you start eating higher quality foods, you won't want to go back to the way you were eating before. Be patient with yourself as you adjust to the diet and realise that your health is on the line – not just your waistline or your thighs. This may be the biggest, most important step you ever make toward self-improvement.

Be patient with yourself as you adjust to the diet and realise that your health is on the line – not just your waistline or your thighs.

After about three weeks, you will start to feel free of the food cravings that have haunted you. After three months, you will be so comfortable with the programme that you won't need to refer to the food lists for guidance – it will all be second nature. After six months, evaluate how well the programme is working for you. Compare your blood glucose, cholesterol and triglyceride levels to your prediet levels. Measure your waist circumference and hips and see if you've lost centimetres. I predict that most of you will have lost a minimum of

5cm (2in) from your problem zone after six months. Once you reach your personal weight and medical targets, you can keep the weight off and remain healthy as long as you stick with the programme.

If you cannot stick with your body shape diet programme for whatever reason, continue to apply the 25 per cent solution to everything you eat. It is the most basic way to cut calories and lose fat.

CHAPTER 11

Apple Shape Diet

M y goals in this chapter are to give you the information you need to:

◆ trim girth from your waist to get rid of dangerous visceral fat;

◆ eat foods that reduce your risk of heart disease, the metabolic syndrome, type 2 diabetes and breast cancer;

◆ improve your overall health and energy as you lose fat; and

◆ break out of diet hell and finally succeed.

If you skipped chapter 10, please go back and read it now. It contains information critical to your success!

Finally, good news for apple-shaped women: trimming girth will be easier for you than it will be for your pear-shaped sisters because visceral fat is the easiest to lose and usually the first to go. Of course, weight loss is much more difficult during and after menopause, regardless of where the fat is deposited. But significant 'waist loss' is certainly within everyone's capability. And don't forget – your immediate goal is to lose only 5cm (2in) from around your waist. That amount of visceral fat loss is often enough to take you out of the disease-risk danger zones.

To help you along, I have created the 'Apple Shape Diet'. If you are currently overweight and want to slim, this programme will help you do that, while also reducing your risks of all the major diseases that plague apple-shaped women. You'll lose subcutaneous fat from other body areas, too, but proportionately more of your fat loss will be from the waist, so your health will begin to improve almost immediately after making dietary changes. If you are not overweight, this programme will help you stay lean and healthy, avoid adding girth to your waist, and give you more vitality than ever before.

Your health will begin to improve almost immediately
after making dietary changes.

The Apple Shape Diet is based on the results of scientific research conducted by top scientists and obesity experts from around the world. These data tell us that, contrary to recent diet fads, carbohydrates are actually good for apple-shaped women – healthy carbohydrates, that is. These healthy or 'Elite' carbs not only help promote weight loss, they can also help lower the risk of cardiovascular disease, the metabolic syndrome and type 2 diabetes. Although this diet can be used by just about anyone, it is especially recommended for apple-shaped women – and the men in their lives, because most men are naturally apple-shaped. Here is what sets this diet plan apart from others:

◆ There is no measuring, weighing or calculating necessary. You'll eat foods by clearly defined categories.

◆ You won't be hungry because there are no limits on the amount of Elite carbs you eat or when you eat them.

◆ You'll have a broader range of foods to choose from, with good, better and best options for flexibility.

◆ This programme addresses the health needs of apple-shaped women throughout their lifespan. There is no need to worry about side effects from the diet or to limit the amount of time you stay on it. If you have high blood pressure, high cholesterol or high blood glucose, this programme will help bring all those measures back into normal range. If you are currently healthy, this programme will ensure that you stay that way.

ELITE FOODS, SUPERIOR DIET

There are only three categories of foods: carbohydrates, fats and proteins. Every food is made up of some combination of just those three macronutrients. There are also vitamins, minerals and phytochemicals, which are also important for vital functions, but they are not foods – they do not provide energy. Carbohydrates, fats and proteins are *all* necessary for the body to function properly. Any diet that tells you to avoid one of these three macronutrients *cannot* be healthy.

Of course, within each macronutrient group, some types of foods are wiser choices than others. The best choices are foods I call Elite carbs, Elite fats or Elite proteins. Elite foods help protect against disease, promote general wellness, and improve your odds of shedding visceral fat. The worst choices are foods I call Wasted carbs, Wasted fats or Wasted proteins. 'Wasted' foods improve your odds of gaining weight, increase your waist size, may act to harm your health and have no redeeming nutritional value. These are the foods that you may have heard others call 'junk food' or 'empty calories'. I prefer the term 'Wasted' because eating them means that you wasted an opportunity to improve your health, and you chose instead to eat something that will contribute to a larger *waist*. Foods that fall somewhere in between –

neither Elite nor Wasted, but healthy enough for a start – I list in columns labelled 'Good' and 'Better'.

WHAT THE APPLE SHAPE DIET LOOKS LIKE

The diet recommendations for apple-shaped women include:

◆ high amounts of Elite carbs;
◆ moderate amounts of Elite fats; and
◆ moderate amounts of Elite proteins.

Unlike many currently popular diet fads, the mainstay of this programme is carbs. Yes, carbs. Many people who want to lose weight have come to believe that carbs are unhealthy – some might say sinfully bad. The message is so pervasive that some restaurants have stopped automatically placing a basket of bread on each table, and people have been avoiding orange juice as if it were battery acid. These are good foods that have been demonised by two main groups: diet gurus who advocate using a low-carbohydrate/high-fat/high-protein weight-loss strategy, and scientists who are proponents of using the glycaemic index to categorise foods. Both groups have championed and popularised the 'carbs are bad' message by exaggerating the significance of their research or beliefs.

Low-Carb Fad Facts

Advocates of low-carbohydrate/high-fat/high-protein diets have helped make carbs the outlaw of the food world. The most controversial and extreme of the carb haters is the Atkins diet, which became popular because people were led to believe that they could eat as much noncarbohydrate food as they wanted. Anything that wasn't a carbohydrate was supposedly fair game, as much as you wanted, any time you wanted it. The 'trick' to the diet was that, at various times, you couldn't eat even healthy carbs, such as wholemeal bread, whole-grain cereal, fruit, beans, rice or pasta. Other low-carb diets have also been popular, but have been less dogmatic in their approaches.

Healthy Elite carbs promote weight loss.

The theory behind these diets is that our bodies rely on carbohydrates for energy. If we don't eat carbohydrates, the body will have to look for energy elsewhere – namely, in fat stores. Plus, the argument goes, carbohydrates raise blood glucose levels, which lead to a rise in insulin, which can lead to storing carbohydrates as fat. So, if you cut out carbohydrates, you won't put on as much fat. This last argument is actually false. Excess calories from all sources are stored as fat – it doesn't matter where they come from. And it is actually harder to store carbohydrates as body fat than it is to store fats as body fat. That's because we need energy (from calories, of course) to convert the carbohydrate food into body fat. Because dietary fat is already in the right form, it takes less energy to convert. What this means for weight gain is that if you eat 1,000 excess calories from carbs, only about 700 of them will be stored as fat. But if you eat 1,000 excess calories from fats, you'll store about 950 of them. So in reality, fat is stored much more efficiently than carbohydrates are.

As a quick weight-loss diet, the Atkins and other low-carbohydrate/high-fat/high-protein plans work, but not because there are any special fat-melting properties in hamburger meat, bacon, cheese and the like. Much of the initial weight loss from low-carb diets comes from the loss of body water. When the last of the body's quick-access stores of carbohydrates are used up, the water that is stored with them is urinated out. This water loss can be easily misinterpreted as weight loss by anyone who steps on some scales. There is also some nonwater weight loss, but that's because the total calorie count is lower, and fewer calories mean weight loss. Even though people are allowed to eat as much fat- and protein-rich foods as they like, it's difficult to eat a lot when you stay away from carbohydrates – a steady diet of steak and eggs gets old pretty quickly.

Because some of the low-carb/high-fat weight-loss reports seemed too good to be true, and because heart specialists were concerned that these high-fat diets might cause heart disease, researchers began looking at how effective and safe the Atkins-type diets are. The results were less than impressive. When different types of diets are compared head-to-head, people on the Atkins-type diets lost more weight in the first six months than people following any other diet. Wait – don't get too excited. After 12 months, everyone ended up losing the same amount of weight, proving that *all diets work equally well in the long run*. That's because calories are the core of weight loss. If you stay on any diet, no matter what its components are, you will lose weight if you cut down on calories.

Safety is another unanswered question. As of this writing, no one has looked at the overall long-term safety of a low-carbohydrate/high-fat/high-protein diet. If these diets actually turn out to be harmful in the long run, a lot of people could end up with major health problems. Short-term studies show that low-carbohydrate diets probably do not harm blood lipid levels, and may actually improve the numbers to some degree, but that is just one measure of health. I'm very concerned with the potential increased risks of type 2 diabetes and cancer. Low-carbohydrate/high-fat diets have been shown to increase the risk of impaired glucose tolerance, and to speed the transition from simple impaired glucose tolerance to outright type 2 diabetes. In the San Luis Valley [Colorado] Diabetes Study, people with impaired glucose tolerance who ate a high-fat diet were more than three times as likely to develop diabetes as those who ate a low-fat diet. We don't know how long this process takes – it probably depends on the individual and her medical history – but if you are trying to lose weight to avoid diabetes, a low-carb/high-fat/high-protein diet does not seem like a wise choice.

Any diet that restricts fruits, grain products, beans or certain vegetables is irresponsible.

Cancer is a whole other potential problem with low-carb diets. Every dietitian and physician knows that eating plenty of fruits and vegetables helps decrease the risk for many types of cancer. Each fruit, vegetable, legume, and grain contains natural *phytochemicals* – 'phyto' meaning 'plant' – that have been shown to prevent or even cure cancer in laboratory animals. There are thousands of phytochemicals, and many of them have the potential to contribute to health in some way. Any diet that restricts fruits, grain products, beans or certain vegetables is irresponsible. Cancer takes 10 to 20 years to develop. My greatest fear is that, in a decade or two, the rate of cancer suddenly will soar and we will realise, too late, that we sacrificed our lives for a low-carb diet fad.

Glycaemic Index

Theoretically, every carbohydrate-based food has its own glycaemic index (GI). Expressed as a number, the GI is a measure of the effects of carbohydrate foods on blood glucose. White bread – with a GI of 100 – is the standard against which all other foods are measured. Other foods have numbers that reflect their relative differences from white bread. For example, the GI of spaghetti is about 45, so it is said to produce less than half the blood glucose response of white bread, making it a 'low-glycaemic' food.

The glycaemic index was originally designed to help people with type 1 diabetes make food choices that would keep blood glucose levels as low as possible. Since then, the use of GI has gained popularity as a diet tool, even though it has never been shown to be effective. And really, when you look closely at the data, there are too many flaws for anyone to use GI realistically or practically. For example, GI cannot be accurately or consistently measured. The GI for any food varies depending on how the food is chosen, cooked, prepared, ripened and even chewed. Some examples: basmati rice has a different GI than American long-grain white rice; a baked potato has a lower GI than a microwaved potato; the GI of a banana increases as it ripens; the GI of a whole potato goes up if you cut it into chunks, and it goes up even higher if you take a fork and mash the chunks. One study even discovered that if you chew your food it will have a higher GI than if you swallow it whole.

All those factors make it very difficult for the average person (or even the exceptionally compulsive person) to use this system to plan a healthy diet. Of course, in the real world, we don't eat individual foods, we tend to eat meals. This complicates the issue of glycaemic index even further. If you eat a high-GI food with a fat- or protein-rich food, the GI goes down. In addition, your glycaemic response to a specific food can vary depending on what time of day you are eating and what foods you ate at the previous meal. That's way too complex for many of us to deal with. I would need some irrefutable evidence that GI seriously impacted my health before I'd want to wade into those murky waters.

That kind of evidence doesn't exist, and for good reason – who could possibly design a realistic study? This is one reason why GI is one of the most hotly contested issues among obesity researchers, dietitians and physicians. There have been a few studies, but the results are conflicting and confusing. The Nurses' Health Study found that women who ate the most high-GI foods had a higher risk of diabetes than those who ate the lowest amounts; but other studies, including the Iowa Women's Health Study, found that glycaemic index, glycaemic load and the total amounts of carbohydrates didn't affect the risk of developing type 2 diabetes at all. In 2004, the American Diabetes Association stated in a published paper that it doesn't support the use of glycaemic index for preventing or treating type 2 diabetes. I prefer to let the nutrition scientists hash out the research. The average person needs a more reliable, real-life solution to the problems of weight loss and healthy eating.

ELITE CARBS AND THE APPLE-SHAPED WOMAN

If you read Part 2 of this book, you know that apple-shaped women have some specific health concerns. Compared with pear-shaped women, they have a higher risk of developing the metabolic syndrome, type 2 diabetes, heart disease and breast cancer. Masses of research has shown that some carbohydrates can be very, very good for us. In the Iowa Women's Health Study, women who ate whole-grain foods often (20 or more servings per week) were found to have a lower risk of developing stroke, heart disease and diabetes than women who ate fewer servings of those foods. In fact, it has been estimated that substituting whole grains for refined grains could reduce the risk of type 2 diabetes by at least 40 per cent. So it really is quite simple: cereal and other whole-grain foods are uniformly found to be great, healthy foods for apple-shaped women. ('Whole grains' means grain-based foods that have not been refined so that they retain much of their natural fibre. Whole wheat, brown rice, oats and barley are the most commonly eaten whole grains. Another way to think about it is that whole grain foods tend to have more of a brown colour, whereas refined grain foods tend to be white – as in white bread and white rice. This programme advocates moving away from white foods and embracing brown foods as healthier and better for your waistline.)

The Apple Shape Diet relies on large amounts of *high-quality* carbohydrates. Carbohydrates are important because they supply the body with glucose. Contrary to common belief, glucose is not, in itself, a bad thing. It only becomes a problem when excess visceral fat causes insulin resistance so that blood glucose builds up to dangerously high levels. Remember, all cells in our bodies need glucose to survive – it is their only energy source. One of the reasons type 2 diabetes is such a dangerous disease is that glucose from the bloodstream can't reach all cells, and without glucose, they die. If enough cells die, organs can fail. Glucose itself is good. High-quality carbohydrates are good. Excess visceral fat is bad.

High-quality carbohydrates help protect against heart disease, cancer and diabetes; they promote gastrointestinal health; and they have been scientifically proven to kick-start weight loss.

High-quality carbohydrates – the Elite carbs – are fruits, vegetables, legumes and whole grains, all of which provide abundant amounts of vitamins, minerals, phytochemicals and fibre, with little or no fat. They help protect against heart disease, cancer and diabetes; they promote gastrointestinal health; and they have been scientifically proven to kick-start weight loss. Want proof? Scientific research tells us that:

◆ A diet high in Elite carbs allows us to eat more food without gaining weight. In studies, people who ate diets high in Elite carbs ended up losing weight – even when they were *encouraged to eat as much as they wanted* within the allotted food choices.

◆ A diet high in Elite carbs can lower insulin response by up to 30 per cent, which can be of considerable importance to apple-shaped women with the metabolic syndrome or type 2 diabetes. In fact, a diet high in Elite carbs has been shown to reduce the risk of developing the metabolic syndrome by about 33 per cent, and type 2 diabetes by up to 45 per cent.

◆ A diet high in Elite carbs can lower low-density lipoprotein (LDL)-cholesterol and triglycerides.

◆ All fruits are Elite carbs. The Women's Health Study showed that women who eat three or more servings of fruit per day can reduce their risk of cardiovascular disease by 43 per cent, compared with women who rarely eat fruit.

◆ All vegetables are Elite carbs. The Women's Health Study showed that women who eat five or more servings of vegetables per day can reduce their risk of cardiovascular disease by 55 per cent, compared with women who rarely eat vegetables.

◆ Elite carbs may make apple-shaped women happier and calmer. Apple-shaped women tend to respond more strongly to intense emotions and psychological states – such as stress, anger and depression – setting up a vicious cycle that leads to more fat building up around the waist. Researchers found that low-carbohydrate diets (like the Atkins diet) seem to make people angrier and more tense and depressed. When stress-prone people eat a high-carbohydrate/ low-protein diet (like the Apple Shape Diet), the effects are reversed. Anger diminishes. They don't feel as depressed. Even the stress-induced cortisol responses decline. So Elite carbs may help apple-shaped women break that cycle of weight gain that comes from stress and anger.

◆ After weight loss, people who eat as much as they want on an Elite carbs diet are more likely to keep weight off than people who follow any other diet plan.

Please keep in mind that all carbohydrates are not the same. While Elite carbs are necessary for life and wellness, there are other carbohydrates that are just a waste. These Wasted carbs include sweets and anything made with white flour – this means virtually all white bread, rolls, baps, hot dog rolls, bagels, muffins (English and American-style), pastries, scones, cakes, biscuits, bread sticks, waffles, pancakes and crackers. Wasted carbs cause kilos and centimetres to pile up, increase your risks for all the apple shape-related diseases, and add virtually nothing to your body except calories.

Fibre – the Lost Puzzle Piece

I grew up hearing my grandmother talk about the importance of 'roughage' for good health. I didn't know exactly what that meant back then, but even in my child-aged mind I knew that I had to eat lots of crispy, leafy, green things in order to have dessert later. Now I realise that my grandmother was wise beyond her years. What was called 'roughage' then is known as 'fibre' now, and it may be an apple-shaped woman's best diet secret.

There are two kinds of fibre: insoluble, which cannot be digested and therefore passes through the body relatively intact (think of the outer shell of a kernel of sweetcorn); and soluble fibre, which dissolves in water. Although both types of fibre seem to be valuable for protecting health, soluble fibre is of particular interest to apple-shaped women. Studies have shown that:

◆ Soluble fibre can lower insulin levels by slowing down digestion and therefore modulating the body's glucose response to food. At relatively high amounts – about 20 grams of fibre per day or more – high blood glucose can be reduced significantly in just 12 weeks.

◆ Eating lots of soluble fibre can protect against heart disease by lowering LDL cholesterol, lowering triglyceride levels, raising HDL cholesterol and reducing blood pressure. Just the simple act of eating more fibre has been shown to decrease the risk of heart attack by 15 per cent.

◆ Both types of fibre are important for weight loss because they make you feel full long after the meal is over, so you eat less in the long run without being hungry.

Elite carbs are high in fibre – either soluble or insoluble, depending on the food. But because fibre is so critical to the health of apple-shaped women, I recommend adding supplemental psyllium, a soluble fibre. The easiest option is to take a psyllium supplement. The most common brands are VitaFiber and Cytoplan/G&G biscuit. Depending on the brand, the supplements are available in capsules or a powder that must be mixed with a beverage. Try to take the supplement immediately before a meal because fibre needs food to work its magic, and always take psyllium supplements with a full glass of water. Don't take a psyllium supplement within two hours of taking medications or other supplements because it may affect their absorption. A small word of warning – as you add fibre to your diet, you may have a little more bloating and flatulence than usual. This is perfectly normal, and the effects will subside after your body adjusts. Note: although it is rare, some people are allergic to psyllium. If you have a history of food allergies, talk with your doctor before trying psyllium.

ELITE FATS AND THE APPLE-SHAPED WOMAN

Our bodies need certain high-quality fats to maintain the structure of cell membranes, regulate blood pressure and maintain the immune system and other functions. In most of the developed nations of the world, getting enough fat isn't a problem. Quite the opposite. We eat plenty of high-fat foods, particularly in the form of hamburgers, French fries, potato crisps, and anything else prepared by frying. Unfortunately, these products contain low-quality fats, the kind that do nothing more than layer more body fat around our waists. Most of us actually eat very little of the high-quality fats that do us any good.

There are three main types of fats: saturated fats, monounsaturated fats and polyunsaturated fats. The word 'saturated' pertains to chemical structure, not to any action on the body or food content.

Saturated Fats

Saturated fats are found in animal products, such as the fat in full-cream milk, cheese, butter, ice cream, lard and the solid fat found in meats. They tend to be solid at room temperature. Palm oil and coconut oil – sometimes called 'tropical oils' on food labels – are also saturated fats. Years and years of data have linked saturated fats to cardiovascular disease and cancer. When people stop eating saturated fats and replace them with mono- or polyunsaturated fats, the risk of heart disease goes down. Because apple-shaped women already have an increased risk of heart disease and cancer, saturated fats pose an extra high threat to them. Therefore, foods high in saturated fats are considered Wasted foods. They should be eaten rarely, if ever.

Monounsaturated Fats

Monounsaturated fats, found primarily in olive oil and rapeseed oil, are among the healthiest fats. Therefore, these are the only oils I recommend for cooking at home. Monounsaturated fats seem to help reduce insulin resistance, making them especially valuable to apple-shaped women with the metabolic syndrome or type 2 diabetes. They also improve blood flow through the arteries, a sign that they may help fight atherosclerosis.

Polyunsaturated Fats

Polyunsaturated fats are divided into three categories:

1. Omega-3 fatty acids. These beneficial fats are found in many kinds of fish, shellfish, rapeseed oil, soyabeans, wheat germ, flaxseed and walnuts. They may help prevent heart attack, hypertension and some forms of cancer, including breast cancer.

2. Omega-6 fatty acids. These are also necessary for good health. Along with omega-3s, omega-6 fats can decrease the inflammation that can contribute to heart disease and type 2 diabetes. Omega-6 is found in meats, corn oil, safflower oil, 'vegetable' oils, leafy vegetables, seeds, nuts and grains.

3. Trans-fatty acids. These are a man-made invention and are just plain dangerous. All *trans* fats are Wasted fats. By taking a polyunsaturated oil and changing the chemical structure, scientists were able to solidify the oil so it could be used for baking and in butter-substitute margarine spreads. The different chemical structure also gives the fat a longer shelf life. Butter and oils go rancid pretty quickly, but trans fats can stay around almost forever. All vending machine baked goods and many store-bought cakes, biscuits and breads contain trans fats, so these products have a double whammy of being high in both Wasted carbs and Wasted fats. The problem is that their altered chemical structure made these fats more dangerous than saturated fats – especially for apple-shaped women. Trans-fatty acids increase the bad LDL cholesterol and decrease the good HDL cholesterol, making heart disease more likely. Eating as little as two tablespoons of a trans-fat margarine a day – either straight or in baked foods – can increase your risk of type 2 diabetes by 25 per cent. This may not seem like much, but Harvard researchers have estimated that the consumption of trans fats causes about 30,000 premature deaths each year in the United States. If you read the ingredient lists on food labels, the words 'partially hydrogenated' mean that oil was turned into a trans fat. Put it back on the shelf. Consumers have become savvy about shopping for products that don't contain trans fats, and manufacturers have responded. Look for labels that say 'No Trans Fats' on bread, biscuits or other baked goods.

Which Fats … and How Much

The fats that are recommended in the Apple Shape Diet are mainly omega-3 fatty acids, omega-6 fatty acids, and monounsaturated fats, with a minimum of saturated fats. No trans fats are recommended – ever. They are virtual poison to apple-shaped women. By lowering the amount of saturated fat in your diet, eliminating trans fats and raising the amounts of omega-3s, you can increase insulin sensitivity and decrease your risk of heart disease – even before you lose a single centimetre.

Apple-shaped women need to eat high-quality, Elite
fats in moderation, rather than either loading up on
high-fat foods or trying to avoid fats.

The Apple Shape Diet allows for a moderate amount of fat, rather than low fat. A study published in a 2004 issue of the *American Journal of Clinical Nutrition* looked at the different effects of a low-fat and a moderate-fat diet on weight loss and health outcomes. Some people ate a low-fat diet in which only 18 per cent of their total calories came from fat, while others ate a moderate-fat diet with 33 per cent of total calories from fat. At the end of the six-week diet and four-week maintenance periods, both groups lost a similar amount of weight. But dieters eating the moderate-fat diet had lower triglyceride levels, with no change in the good HDL cholesterol. Those on a low-fat diet, however, had no decrease in triglycerides and an unhealthy decrease in HDL cholesterol. This means that apple-shaped women need to eat high-quality, Elite fats in moderation, rather than either loading up on high-fat foods or trying to avoid fats.

Although fish and olive oils are the top recommended fats, they won't usually taste too good on your breakfast toast. The good news for apple-shaped women is that manufacturers have developed margarine-like spreads from a soyabean extract, which contain no trans-fatty acids. These spreads, such as Benecol, inhibit the absorption of cholesterol from the small intestine. After just two weeks of using them instead of regular margarine or butter, the dangerous LDL cholesterol levels can be reduced by up to 14 per cent. That's rather impressive, considering it simply requires changing your bread spread. These spreads can also be used for baking or sautéing, so you can reduce the amounts of harmful fats in other home-cooked meals as well. These spreads cost more than margarine or butter, but you may end up saving money in the long run if you don't need to buy a cholesterol-lowering prescription.

Another Look at Nuts

Nuts are unique in the food world. They are high in carbohydrate, fat, protein and fibre – all of the Elite variety – which makes nuts an all-around smart choice for apple-shaped women. I've included them as a fat because they cannot be eaten in large quantities the way Elite carbs can, and their greatest health benefits seem to come from the types of oil they contain. In the Nurses' Health Study, women who ate 30g (1oz) of nuts on most days of the week lowered their risk of heart disease by 35 per cent. Among women with diabetes, the effect was even greater, with risk of heart disease lowered by 47 per cent. Walnuts contain relatively high amounts of omega-3 fatty acids, which have additional heart-healthy effects. There is also some evidence that nuts and peanut butter may lower the risk of type 2 diabetes by up to 25 per cent.

There's something special about nuts. When people incorporate nuts into their diets, their weight has a tendency to go down even if they make no other changes in their diets.

Even more important for apple-shaped women is that eating nuts seems to help you lose weight, almost magically. Yes, the fats and fibre in nuts help fill you up and keep you satisfied longer than most other foods, but there's something special about nuts. When people incorporate nuts into their diets, their weight has a tendency to go down. Nuts seem to defy the normal expectations for weight gain. For example, when people in studies were forced to eat a certain amount of nuts – an amount that, according to the calorie calculations, should have made them gain a considerable amount of weight, they gained much less than expected. The trick is to limit yourself to about 30g (1oz) of nuts per day. That's about 28 peanuts, 14 walnut halves, 22 almonds, 20 pecan halves or two tablespoons of peanut butter. If you can't stop at 30g (1oz), limit yourself to a total of 200g (7oz) of nuts per week – more than that and you *will* gain weight, and there are no additional health benefits.

ELITE PROTEINS
AND THE APPLE-SHAPED WOMAN

Proteins provide the building blocks that allow us to repair damage in our bodies, build a strong immune system, make hormones and blood cells, develop muscle and generally stay healthy. All proteins are made up of chains of molecules called amino acids. There are about 20 different amino acids necessary for good health – 11 that our bodies make themselves, and 9 (called the 'essential' amino acids) that we can only get from food. Different food sources contain different amino acids, therefore we usually need to eat more than one type of protein food to get all the dietary protein our bodies need. Most people in the developed countries eat more than enough protein, so getting enough isn't usually a problem. As with fats, quality is the issue.

Protein is found in a wide variety of food sources, including eggs, meat, poultry, fish, dairy products, whole grains, beans and nuts. Elite proteins are those that provide a good amino acid balance with no saturated fat. These include soyabean products, kidney beans, chickpeas, pinto beans, rolled oats, lentils, nuts, egg whites and whole wheat. Whole eggs contain too much cholesterol to be considered Elite proteins, but they are no longer considered off-limits, even to people with high cholesterol levels. Dietitians generally agree that people who eat a minimal amount of saturated fats can safely eat up to one egg a day. Wasted proteins are those that contain a lot of saturated fats and therefore are likely to raise cholesterol and increase the risk for heart disease. These include many types of red meat, processed meats and cheese.

SOYA FOODS

Many of the Elite proteins recommended in the Apple Shape Diet are soyabean based, which means that they are also Elite carbs. The world has known about the joys of soya products for thousands of years, but Western countries are just beginning to catch on. The soyabean has the highest quality protein possible for a vegetable, containing nearly all the amino acids we need in a highly digestible form. Although the only time most of us use the word 'soya' is in conjunction with the word 'sauce', soyabean products are extremely tasty, satisfying, and healthy – if you can get past the word.

The Psychology of Soya

The American food psychologist Dr. Brian Wansink and his colleagues conducted an intriguing study of how people respond to the word 'soy'. People were asked to participate in a taste test of a new nutrition bar. Although all participants tasted the same product, they saw one of four different labels that had different health messages: (1) 'Contains 10 grams soy protein'; (2) 'Contains 10 grams protein'; (3) 'May help reduce the risk of heart disease'; and (4) no health claim. After tasting the nutrition bar, the subjects were asked to rate its taste, texture and flavour. In reality, the nutrition bar contained no soya protein at all, so any difference in taste ratings between the label marked 'soy' and the other labels would be due entirely to preconceived notions of soya, not to any actual taste differences. The researchers found that people who did not generally consider themselves 'health conscious' rated the bar marked 'soy' much worse than the bars with other labels. They thought the soya protein bar looked worse, tasted worse, they didn't enjoy eating it and they had no intention of buying it. The other bars – the exact same food but without the word 'soy' on the label – were rated much higher. The bar that was rated the best was the bar with the label that contained no health claims at all.

We expect healthy food to taste bad, and we adjust our taste buds accordingly. If we think it's good for us, we won't like it. If we ever want to change our eating patterns, we have to fight our psychology.

This tells us that we expect healthy food to taste bad, and we adjust our taste buds accordingly. If we think it's good for us, we won't like it. We won't even like the way it *looks*, even if it isn't what we think it is. The first lesson is that if we ever want to change our eating patterns, we have to fight our psychology. Just knowing that this bias occurs will help you to recognise your own food prejudices and to approach new foods with an open mind.

The second lesson is that if you are trying to introduce a new food to your family, for heaven's sake don't tell them what it is. Don't even tell them that it is healthy. When they ask, be creative. Make something up. Tell them that it is a new product line from their favourite frozen-food manufacturer. If you say that it's good for them, they won't give it a chance.

Health Benefits of Soya

Keeping that in mind, here's what we know about soya products:

◆ Eating soya foods may help premenopausal women reduce their risk of breast cancer by about 34 per cent.

◆ Eating soya foods may help all women reduce their risk of endometrial cancer by about 33 per cent.

◆ Researchers believe that soya can help people lose weight and control or prevent diabetes by reducing insulin resistance, improving glucose tolerance and increasing insulin sensitivity. People with type 2 diabetes who eat soya foods seem to be able to maintain better control over their blood sugar.

◆ Eating soya foods reduces the risk of heart disease by lowering cholesterol, reducing blood pressure and improving vascular reactivity. Switching from animal protein (meats and dairy foods) to soya protein in your diet can lower cholesterol by up to 24 per cent.

◆ Postmenopausal women who eat more soya foods tend to have a smaller waist circumference than women who don't eat soya foods. We don't know whether this is due to the benefit of isoflavones and other phytochemicals in soya, or to the low-calorie, low-fat nature of soya foods. Still, the correlation exists, and I'm all for anything that might possibly help reduce the health risks for apple-shaped women.

These positive effects come only from soya foods, not from isolated phytochemicals, such as isoflavones. Soya supplements don't work – you have to eat the foods. In fact, the pure isolates found in soya supplements may even be harmful in large doses, but it is impossible to overdose on soya compounds when eaten in foods.

Tasty Ways to Add Soya Foods to Your Diet

◆ **Meat substitutes.** The easiest way to add soya foods to your diet is to try the meat-substitute products – especially the Morningstar Farms brand products – found in the freezer section of health food stores and some supermarkets. The most familiar soya-based frozen food is the veggie burger, which has become so popular that it has made its way onto some restaurant menus. But there is a full range of soya bean-based frozen meat substitutes that taste remarkably close to the real thing. You can find substitute chicken cutlets and nuggets, turkey slices, sausage, hot dogs, paté, streaky bacon and fish cakes.

◆ **Tempeh.** This soya food comes in blocks that are about the size of a television remote control, usually found in the chilled section of supermarket produce departments. The easiest way to enjoy tempeh is to cut the block into 1cm (½in), bite-sized pieces, then marinate them in the same sauce you would use to marinate chicken or beef. Simply put the marinade and tempeh bits in a covered container or resealable plastic bag, shake to distribute the sauce, then put it in the refrigerator for at least an hour, up to 24 hours. (If marinating longer than one hour, shake the container periodically.) Then sauté the bits in two tablespoons of olive oil until the surfaces are browned. Serve over rice or other grain, use as a taco filling or mix into a casserole. If you have any left over, refrigerate them and use as a substitute for croutons in salad. When tempeh is prepared in this manner, most people can't tell that they are not eating meat.

◆ **Tofu.** Tofu is soya bean curd, with a consistency similar to cottage cheese. It can be marinated and prepared in the same manner as tempeh, but it won't brown – it just needs to be heated through. Silken tofu is much softer, about the consistency of soured cream, and can be substituted for soured cream in dips and other recipes. Start by substituting silken tofu for half the soured cream in any recipe to adjust to the slightly different taste, or add more seasoning to the dip to mask the change.

◆ **Soya milk.** Soya milk is a beverage made from pressed soyabeans. It is available in several flavours, including vanilla, chocolate and 'original'. If you are trying soya milk for the first time, opt for one of the flavours because many people find original soya milk less pleasing initially. Let's just say it's an acquired taste. On the other hand, vanilla and chocolate flavours taste more like drinking a very thin milkshake. Soya milk can be substituted for regular milk in recipes, and it is terrific over cereal or in fruit smoothies. One die-hard, anti-soya person I know was finally swayed when she discovered that chocolate soya milk in her coffee was even better than creamer. Always buy the fortified soya milk, which has added calcium, vitamin D and vitamin B_{12}.

◆ **Soya butter.** Soya butter is just like peanut butter, but with a slightly sweeter taste. Look for varieties that contain no added oils or sweeteners. Soya butter can be found in health food stores, organic markets and some of the larger supermarkets.

Most of these soya products are so popular that they are carried by supermarkets, as well as health food stores. Remember – keep an open mind and try not to let preconceived notions of soya keep you from becoming healthier and leaner.

THE APPLE SHAPE DIET PROGRAMME

Important note for people with type 2 diabetes: if you follow the Apple Shape Diet, there is a good chance that your blood glucose levels will be lower than usual. Monitor your blood glucose levels more closely to make sure that you adjust your medication or insulin properly. If you see dramatic changes, talk with your doctor, discuss your programme, and confirm that your treatment plan is still optimal. Some people with type 2 diabetes who take oral medication or insulin may be able to reduce their dose or go off insulin entirely if their blood glucose levels come under better control.

Now that you understand the principles behind the recommendations, the basics of the Apple Shape Diet are simple:

1. You can eat as many Elite carbs and Elite proteins as you want. For any meal, for any snack, if you eat Elite foods then you don't have to weigh, measure or count anything. Of course, use common sense about portions. This is not a prescription for gorging yourself, even if the foods are healthy. It's just that you don't have to measure out half a cup of brown rice or count out 12 grapes. Simply eat a satisfying amount. Too much of anything will cause you to gain weight.

2. Substitute Elite fats for the oils and spreads you currently use. Do not increase how often you eat fats, just make a simple substitution to avoid adding extra calories in your diet. In the diet, nuts are considered a fat only because they need to be limited. Incorporate nuts into your diet as snacks or as meal ingredients, but aim to eat no more than 200 grams (7oz) of nuts each week.

3. To slim faster, keep applying the 25 per cent solution. I would rather have you stick to the diet than to cut calories in the beginning, but if you can do both, you'll be better off.

4. Avoid all products listed in the 'Wasted' columns for all food groups and meals. If you cannot avoid them entirely, cut down as much as possible.

5. Foods listed in the columns marked 'Good' and 'Better' need to be eaten infrequently and in limited amounts. Every day, limit yourself to no more than two Good choices and three Better choices. This means that throughout the day, you are allowed to eat up to five portions of foods not listed as an Elite food. If you prefer, you may substitute a Better choice for a Good choice.

6. For Good and Better foods, think of a portion as a single unit (one bagel, one container of yoghurt, one pork chop, one egg) or the amount you would have eaten before the diet (the same number of slices of turkey on your sandwich, the same amount of breakfast cereal). So, for example, if you decide to eat a wholewheat bagel, one bagel is one serving. If you have two wholewheat bagels, that counts as two of your five Good/Better foods.

7. If you decide to eat a Wasted food, try to follow the 'Limit the Damage' rules outlined below. Your next two meals should contain nothing but Elite foods – nothing from the Good, Better or Wasted categories. So if you eat doughnuts for breakfast, your lunch and dinner choices need to be only Elite foods.

8. Eat three meals and three snacks each day. It is OK to skip a snack, but it is never OK to skip a meal – it just sets you up for overeating later in the day.

Limit the Damage

People are not perfect, and following a diet is difficult, so we are bound to 'cheat' every once in a while. I recognise this, and I want you to know that a little controlled cheating is expected. All I ask is that you try to limit the damage:

◆ If possible, wait until the weekend. Try to reserve one day that is your 'cheating day' for the week. Get it out of your system then, and eat Elite the rest of the week.

◆ Instead of a Wasted food, try to find a substitute in the Good or Better food categories.

◆ Don't let a Wasted food go down alone. Have a psyllium fibre supplement, a wholemeal bread or a green salad immediately before you eat a Wasted food. The fibre will delay the absorption of the carbohydrate to balance out its effects on blood sugar and will slow stomach emptying so you'll feel full longer.

◆ If you plan to eat a very sweet Wasted food, try to eat an Elite carb or an Elite protein beforehand – this may limit the rush of glucose that will make your energy crash in an hour or two.

◆ Look for ways to make your choices smarter. If you are determined to eat a slab of white bread with butter and jam, ask yourself if multigrain or wholemeal bread would do as well, or if you could substitute an Elite spread for the butter. Every food decision is important.

Breakfast

◆ **Eat breakfast every day.** Many women who are trying to lose weight skip breakfast. They feel that it is easier just to run straight to work or get on with the tasks of the day than it is to think about a healthy breakfast. Plus, there's that myth that if you only eat two meals a day, you will eat one-third fewer calories, so you'll lose weight. Not true. Studies have shown that people who eat breakfast are about half as likely to be obese as people who don't eat breakfast. Additional bonus: eating breakfast seems to help reduce insulin resistance, which means a lower risk of developing type 2 diabetes. We don't know if this is simply because breakfast eaters are less hungry later in the day, or if there is some hormonal effect related to blood glucose levels. Either way, breakfast is a smart choice. It's important for apple-shaped women to know that breakfast in general causes the highest rise in blood glucose, therefore it is especially important not to eat Wasted foods for breakfast.

Note: The choices in the following charts are suggestions based on typical foods eaten at these particular meals. There is no reason why you could not eat whole wheat spaghetti for breakfast, or a psyllium-based breakfast cereal for dinner.

Breakfast Choices

WASTED	GOOD	BETTER	ELITE
White flour foods	Eggs	Peanut butter	Whole fruit – any kind
White bread	Back bacon	Soya butter	Wholemeal bread
Muffins	Dried fruits	Nuts	Multigrain bread
Cinnamon rolls	Baked goods that are whole-grain and contain no trans fats	Low-fat yoghurt	Rye bread
Most bagels		Cottage cheese	Pumpernickel bread
American style muffins		Skimmed milk	Porridge
Danish pastry	Homemade American-style muffins	Unsweetened muesli	Cereals
Doughnuts	Wholegrain or fruit		Wholegrain
Scones			Egg whites
Croissants	Wholewheat pancakes		Meat substitutes
Brioches			Bacon (soya)
Pancakes	Fruit juice		Sausages (soya)
Pain au chocolat	Semi-skimmed milk		
Sugary breakfast cereal	Jam or marmalade		
Fried potatoes			

WASTED	GOOD	BETTER	*ELITE*
Any kind of sausage	Honey		Benecol spread
Streaky bacon			Coffee
Butter			Tea
Most margarine			Green tea
Full cream milk			Soya milk
Cream			
Cola drinks			
Sports drinks			
'Diet' drinks			

Suggestions . . .

◆ Wholemeal toast with peanut butter or soya butter. Add jam, marmalade, or honey to use one Good food.

◆ Whole-grain cereal with soya milk. Add berries or bananas. (All unlimited.)

◆ Soya-milk smoothie, made by blending vanilla soya milk with your choice of fruit. My favourite is half a banana with a cup of blueberries, strawberries or raspberries.

◆ Porridge with a dollop of yoghurt or Elite spreads. Add berries, banana or other fresh whole fruit. (All unlimited . . . a small amount of yoghurt won't count as a limited food.) Add nuts.

◆ Cottage cheese or yoghurt (one Better food) with fruit. Add a touch of honey to use a Good food. Add some nuts.

◆ Hardboiled or scrambled eggs (uses one or two Good foods), with wholemeal toast. Or, an egg-white omelette with diced tomatoes, mushrooms and peppers (unlimited). Or, an egg-white omelette with a filling of soya-based bacon substitute (unlimited).

◆ Homemade wholemeal or fruit muffins are allowable under the Good category if made with the Elite spreads, olive oil or rapeseed oil.

◆ Fruit juice is actually healthy for you. Although there has been a lot of anti-juice propaganda coming from the fad diet groups, fruit juice contains a high quantity of antioxidant vitamins. Orange juice may help lower the risk of heart disease by improving elasticity of blood vessels after a fatty meal. It does contain a lot of natural sugars and calories, so it is fattening in large quantities – that's why you can't have unlimited quantities. Fruit juice is included here in the Good category.

◆ Feel free to drink coffee or tea. People with type 2 diabetes used to be told not to drink coffee because it was thought to worsen glycaemic control. Research published in 2004 showed that women who drink three to four cups of coffee per day have about a 30 per cent lower risk of developing type 2 diabetes than women who drink less than three cups per day. Further, women who drink five or more cups of coffee per day lower their risk of diabetes by an amazing 60 per cent. (Keep in mind that even a medium-sized mug holds more than one cup of coffee. A large mug can hold three cups.) Black tea (the usual type found in packaged tea bags) and green tea reduce total and LDL cholesterol and may stimulate weight loss. Green tea leaf is used in traditional Chinese medicine as a treatment for obesity, and habitual tea drinkers tend to have less body fat and a smaller waist circumference than non-tea drinkers.

◆ **Take a multivitamin with breakfast.** No one eats a perfectly balanced diet all the time. In order to catch all the necessary nutrients, I recommend taking a multivitamin every day. In addition, you'll reduce your risk of colorectal cancer by about 30 per cent and heart disease by about 25 per cent. The supplement you choose should supply 400 micrograms of folic acid (folate), 400 IU vitamin D, 6 micrograms vitamin B_{12}, and 3 milligrams vitamin B_6. Premenopausal women also need 15 milligrams of iron. After menopause, taking additional iron in a supplement may actually contribute to heart disease. My personal favourite multivitamins for premenopausal women are regular Centrum. For postmenopausal women I recommend Centrum Select 50+. Some people just have a hard time swallowing pills. For them, I recommend looking for chewable children's vitamins. Believe it or not, chewing just one is great for premenopausal women. Postmenopausal women can chew *two* tablets which do not contain iron.

◆ **Take a psyllium supplement.** Although you can take psyllium any time during the day, I recommend that you take it in the morning so that it can do its magic while your body is active. If you find that the supplement gives you too much flatulence if you take it early, feel free to take it later in the day.

◆ **Take two 500-milligram calcium supplements each day.** It is extremely difficult for women to get enough calcium from diet alone. Although apple-shaped women don't usually have a problem with osteoporosis, you still want to keep your bone density at its highest level. Calcium has two quirks. First, it takes up a lot of space. No multivitamin can offer the full 1,000 milligrams necessary because the pill would be too big to swallow, so you have to take a separate supplement. Second, our bodies can only absorb 500 milligrams of calcium at a time, so we have to take the pills at different times of the day. In medical terms, this is called a divided dose. I recommend taking one 500-milligram tablet with lunch, and a second with dinner. Taking the supplements with meals ensures that they are absorbed properly. Don't pay extra for fancy oyster shell or coral calcium – they are no better than regular calcium, and oyster shell supplements can contain contaminants, such as lead. The only time I think paying a little extra is worth it is if you want to turn calcium supplements into a treat. The chewable Ellactiva calcium supplements are available in two flavours, caramel and strawberry. It makes remembering to take your vitamins a joy – and because sweets are on the Wasted list for apple-shaped women, here's your chance to get your guilt-free treats two times a day.

Midmorning

◆ **Eat a midmorning snack if you are hungry.**

◆ **Always carry an Elite carb snack in your handbag or briefcase.** If you are not prepared, you may be tempted to buy vending machine food, all of which is to be avoided. But if you have a snack plan, you'll be less likely to be seduced by unhealthy food in a moment of weakness.

Snack Choices			
WASTED	**GOOD**	**BETTER**	***ELITE***
White flour foods	Dried fruits	Nuts	Whole fruit – any kind
White bread	Baked goods that are whole-grain and contain no trans fats	Peanut or soya butter	Vegetables
Most muffins, English or American		Wholemeal crackers	Wholemeal bread
Cinnamon rolls	Homemade cookies	Yoghurt	Multigrain bread
Most bagels	Oatmeal-raisin	Yoghurt dressing	Rye bread
Danish pastry	Baked potato crisps	Cottage cheese	Pumpernickel bread
Doughnuts		Ice lolly	Legumes
Scones	Baked corn chips	Skimmed milk	Whole-grain cereal
Popcorn, with butter	Plain digestive biscuits	(virtually) No-fat cream cheese	Coffee
Chips	Soya pretzels	(virtually) No-fat fromage frais	Tea
Potato crisps, regular	Rice cakes		Green tea
	Popcorn, no butter		Soya milk
	Frozen yoghurt		Tofu dressing
	Fruit juice		Olive oil dressing

WASTED	GOOD	BETTER	*ELITE*
Corn chips, regular	Semi-skimmed milk		
Pretzels, regular	Jam or marmalade		
Ice cream	Honey		
Sweets	Low-fat mayonnaise		
Cream salad dressings	Cheese		
Full cream milk			
Cream			
Cola drinks			
Sports drinks			
'Diet' drinks			

Suggestions . . .

◆ Sliced or baby carrots, celery stalks, red pepper wedges, cucumber slices, courgette sticks or broccoli florets with a yoghurt or tofu dressing dip.

◆ Sprinkle whole-grain cereal into a cup of yoghurt.

◆ Three-bean salad with an olive oil and vinegar dressing.

◆ Fruit salad, alone or with yoghurt. Fresh fruit is best, frozen fruit is next best. If you are really in a time pinch, you can use tinned fruit salad – but only if it doesn't contain syrup.

◆ Soya pretzels with a mustard dip.

◆ Wholemeal crackers with cheese or peanut butter . . . or, even better, with a tofu or no-fat cream cheese spread (made by blending a soft tofu or cream cheese with your choice of fruit, herbs or vegetables). Make sure the crackers don't contain *trans* fats.

◆ The new 'low-carb' snack foods are not good substitutes for the healthy Elite carbs recommended here. I can tell you from experience that the majority of prepared low-carb foods don't taste very good, and they are very expensive. Worst of all, they are little more than a marketing scheme to take advantage of the low-carb fad. One of the reasons that low-carb diets work at all is that they limit food choices so that you eat less. If you start eating low-carb ice cream, biscuits, pasta, cereal and other products, you'll end up eating unnecessary calories and gaining weight eventually. The goal should be to get into the lifelong habit of eating healthy foods – not the latest processed foods to match the diet of the day.

Lunch

◆ **Prepare your own lunch so that you can control the ingredients.** Eating lunch out is a trial when you are trying to eat healthy foods. The world conspires to make you choose Wasted foods, or to get you to overeat. If you bring your own lunch to work or have something handy at home, you'll be less tempted to eat fast food.

Lunch Choices			
WASTED	**GOOD**	**BETTER**	*ELITE*
Anything fried Anything made with trans fats White flour foods 　White bread 　Hot dog roll 　Bap	Baked goods that are whole-grain and contain no trans fats Ham Hard cheese 　Cheddar 　Swiss	Nuts Peanut and soya butter Wholemeal crackers Yoghurt Yoghurt dressing Chicken	Whole fruit – any kind Vegetables, except potato Salad (vegetable) Wholemeal bread Rye bread

WASTED	GOOD	BETTER	ELITE
Breadsticks	Provolone	Turkey	Pumpernickel bread
Cheese rolls	Sirloin steak	Fish*	Multigrain bread
French bread	T-bone steak	Tuna	Soya products
Hot dogs	Dried fruits	Swordfish	Veggie burgers
Beef hamburger	Pitta	Soft cheese	Veggie hot dogs
Cornish pasty	Potato	Feta	Legumes, lentils
Fried chicken	Baked potato crisps	Goat's cheese	Wholewheat pasta
Polish sausage	Baked corn chips	Cottage cheese	Tagliatelle verdi
Salami	Soya pretzels	Wholemeal pitta	Fish*
Pastrami	Rice cakes	Ice lolly	Salmon
Bologna	Popcorn, no butter	Skimmed milk	Cod
Corned beef	Frozen yoghurt	No-fat soured cream	Halibut
Chorizo	Fruit juice	Shellfish	Trout
Spareribs	Semi-skimmed milk		Hummus
Bacon	Jam or marmalade		Olive oil dressing
Corn chips, regular	Honey	*Tuna, swordfish, shark and marlin are not Elite because they tend to contain high levels of mercury, which can be harmful if eaten in large quantities. Women who are pregnant, breast-feeding or trying to conceive should eat no more than two medium-sized tins of tuna, or one tuna steak, per week. Pregnant women, infants and children under 16 years of age should avoid eating shark, swordfish and marlin.	Coffee
Pretzels, regular	Low-fat mayonnaise		Tea
Ice cream			Green tea
Cream dressings			Soya milk
Full cream milk			Tofu dressing
Cream			
Sweets			
Cola drinks			
Sports drinks			
'Diet' drinks			

Suggestions . . .

◆ Veggie burger on wholemeal toast, topped with your favourite hamburger toppings.

◆ Soya-based chicken rissole with tomato sauce and a sprinkling of feta cheese.

◆ Hummus on wholemeal bread or pitta, topped with roasted red pepper and/or Kalamata olive bits.

◆ Salmon mayonnaise sandwich. When we think of fish for lunch, many of us automatically think of tuna salad. Really, any fish can be turned into a tasty spread, and salmon is one of my favourites. Try mixing tinned salmon with a dollop of low-fat mayonnaise, sultanas, walnuts and finally chopped celery, and serving it in a pitta or on wholemeal bread.

◆ Elite chicken sandwich spread. Dice the meat from a roasted chicken (store-bought if you are in a hurry), and mix with celery, walnuts, halved red grapes (or other favourite combinations). Add two tablespoons olive oil and one tablespoon lemon juice, and mix thoroughly. The olive oil is an Elite substitute for mayonnaise, and makes a lighter-tasting spread. Put on wholemeal bread for a sandwich, or serve on a bed of greens to make a salad.

Afternoon Snack

◆ **Eat an afternoon snack if you are hungry.** This snack is what I call the 'excuse snack'. We may not be hungry, but it's a great excuse to take a break from work, or sit down with the kids after school, or procrastinate before making dinner or starting some other evening project. Resolve to make this snack as healthy as possible so that you know you are eating from hunger and not from boredom or another excuse. If you are not hungry enough to eat something healthy, then maybe you don't need the snack. Use the same snack list as for the midmorning snack.

Dinner

◆ **Don't forget to take your second calcium supplement.**

Dinner Choices			
WASTED	**GOOD**	**BETTER**	*ELITE*
Anything fried	Baked goods – only if whole-grain and contain no trans fats	Nuts	Whole fruit – any kind
Anything made with trans fats		Peanut and soya butter	Vegetables, not fried
White flour foods	Ham	Wholemeal crackers	Salad (vegetable)
White bread	Hard cheese:	Pasta, regular	Wholemeal bread
Hot dog roll	Cheddar	Wild rice	Pumpernickel bread
Bap	Red Leicester	Chicken	Rye bread
Breadsticks	Stilton	Turkey	Multigrain bread
Crusty rolls	Swiss	Venison	Corn tortillas
Cheese rolls	Potato/root vegetable	Buffalo/bison meat	Soya products
French bread	Sirloin steak	Fish	Veggie burgers
Ciabatta	T-bone steak	Tuna	Veggie hot dogs
Hot dogs	Roast pork leg	Swordfish	Meat substitutes
Beef hamburger	Pork shoulder	Shellfish	Tempeh
Fried chicken	Pork chops	Oysters, clams	Tofu
Polish sausage	Egg noodles	Mussels	Legumes, lentils
Salami	White rice	Soft cheese:	Wholewheat pasta
Pastrami	Couscous	Feta	Tagliatelle verdi
Bologna	Pitta, regular	Goat's cheese	Brown rice
Corned beef	Flour tortilla	Cottage cheese	
Chorizo	Polenta	Wholemeal pitta	
Spareribs	Low-fat mayonnaise	Olives	
Bacon		Yoghurt	
Spam			

WASTED	GOOD	BETTER	*ELITE*
Duck		(virtually) No-fat cream cheese	Bulgar wheat
Goose		(virtually) No-fat fromage frais	Wheat berries
Panfried pork chops		Yogurt dressing	Quinoa
Lamb			Barley
Veal			Fish
Cream dressings			Salmon
			Cod
			Halibut
			Trout
			Tomato sauce
			Hummus
			Olive oil dressing
			Tofu dressing

Suggestions . . .

◆ Become creative with old recipes. Start to substitute Elite foods for any Wasted foods you currently include in your diet. Dinner is a great time to experiment because there are so many Elite options to choose from. For example, substitute chickpeas or soya-based meatless mince for beef mince in casseroles and chilli. Diced and sautéed portobello mushrooms also make a good meat substitute. Start to substitute wholewheat pasta for regular pasta, brown rice for white rice – if the taste is too strong, try mixing the old with the new. (They have to be prepared separately because their cooking times are different, but you can mix them on the plate. See Elite Grains page 248.)

◆ Learn to sauté. One of the basic tricks of the healthy kitchen is to heat two tablespoons of olive oil in a frying pan over medium-high heat. Then, add any combination of vegetables you like – in order of 'toughness' – giving each new level two to five minutes of individual cooking time. First add onions and garlic, then the stalky vegetables (broccoli, celery, cauliflower), then the firm vegetables (red or green peppers, carrots), then mushier vegetables (olives, artichoke hearts), and finally the leafy vegetables (spinach, kale). Use your imagination; play around with different combinations. Serve over a whole grain or pasta.

Whole-Grain Preparation

ELITE Grains

Whole-grain foods are more flavourful than refined grains. Many people find that after a few servings of whole grains they no longer enjoy the plain, bland white rice or regular pasta. The basic preparation is the same – bring water to a boil, add the grain, reduce heat, cover the pot and simmer until done. Only the grain-to-water ratio and cooking time change. Tip: you can have an even tastier grain if you substitute chicken or vegetable broth for water in the following instructions.

◆ **Bulgar wheat** is granulated wheat and looks like chopped-up rice. It has a slightly richer flavour than brown rice, and can be used exactly as you would use rice – as a base for stir-fry, with chilli, or as a side dish. Bulgar wheat is found in many supermarkets. To prepare: Use two cups water to one cup bulgar; simmer, covered, for 15 minutes.

◆ **Brown rice** is a nice, mild grain that has become popular in Britain in recent years. It is more satisfying, more flavourful, and has about three times the fibre as white rice. Brown rice is available in all supermarkets. To prepare: use two cups water to one cup brown rice; simmer, covered, for about 40 minutes or until all the water is absorbed.

◆ **Quinoa** (pronounced KEEN-wah) is an ancient grain that provides all the amino acids we need, making it a complete protein. It is a light grain in looks, weight and taste. It can be used in place of rice as a side dish, or as a base to a lighter topping, such as sautéed vegetables with marinated tempeh. Quinoa is available in health food stores. To prepare: quinoa needs to be rinsed thoroughly before cooking. Use two cups water to one cup quinoa; simmer, covered, for about 15 to 20 minutes.

◆ **Wheat berries** are the whole whole wheat. It is how all other wheat products start out. This is the purest form of wheat. Wheat berries have a nutty flavour that everyone seems to love. The main drawback is the long cooking time. Still, if you prepare a large batch of wheat berries, they can be frozen and saved for whenever you choose to eat them. They are found in health food stores and organic markets. To prepare: Use four cups of water to one cup of wheat berries; simmer for about three hours. (Not all the water will be absorbed.)

Desserts

As a physician, I am not in favour of anyone eating dessert (except for fruit, of course). However, as a human being, I know that I can't always resist sweet foods. My recommendation is to eat desserts only on the weekends. If you normally eat something sweet every day, the weekend dessert plan will cut your sweets consumption by about two-thirds. Whenever possible, try to eat Good, Better or Elite desserts. They will give you a taste of something yummy without going overboard on Wasted calories.

Remember, most store-bought baked goods are full of *trans*-fatty acids, the worst things an apple-shaped woman can eat. If a chocolate chip cookie or a slice of cake is in your future, I would much rather it be one that you make yourself at home. The best baked goods use applesauce or prune purée instead of butter (these can be substituted for butter measure-for-measure). Next best would be to bake using one of the Elite spreads (such as Benecol) or extra-light olive oil, which doesn't have the distinctive olive oil taste or aroma. The spreads can be substituted measure-for-measure. If you choose to use olive oil, use one-quarter less olive oil than butter – instead of using 225g (8oz) of butter, you should use 170ml (6fl oz) of olive oil. And of course, anytime you can add dried or fresh fruit or nuts to a dessert recipe, it will be healthier.

Dessert Choices			
WASTED	**GOOD**	**BETTER**	*ELITE*
White flour foods	Dried fruits	Sorbet	Whole fruit – any kind
Most gâteau/cakes	Homemade biscuits	Ice lolly	Applesauce
Most American-style muffins	Homemade cake	Frozen yogurt	Soya-milk smoothie
Danish pastry	Fruit tart	Chocolate-covered nuts	
Doughnuts	Fruit crumbles	Oatmeal-raisin cookies	
Scones		Hard muesli bars	
Cupcakes			
Most biscuits/cookies			
Non-fruit tarts			
Sweets			
Ice cream			

Evening snack

◆ **Eat an evening snack if you need to.** This is the most optional of all the snacks. My usual recommendation is not to eat anything after 8 P.M., but I understand that this habit can be difficult to break. Use the same snack list as for the midmorning snack.

◆ **If you have heart disease, remember the fish oil.** As described in chapter 6, people with heart disease can benefit from taking fish oil supplements. On days when you don't eat fish, take 1,000 milligrams of fish oil in capsule form. All brands seem to be equal in quality, so choose the one you are most comfortable with, either in terms of price or brand. (Always check with your doctor before starting to take fish oil supplements. Because fish oil thins the blood, it usually isn't recommended if you have a bleeding disorder, or if you are already taking a blood-thinning medication, such as warfarin.) I make this recommendation here because many people find that they don't suffer from fishy breath quite so badly if they take the supplements at night.

CHAPTER 12

Pear Shape Diet

My goals in this chapter are to give you the information you need to:

◆ avoid excess weight gain that can transform your body into an apple shape;

◆ understand what it takes to lose fat from your pear zone;

◆ eat foods that will reduce your risk of osteoporosis;

◆ improve your overall health and energy as you lose fat;

◆ break out of diet hell, and finally succeed.

If you skipped chapter 10, please go back and read it now. It contains information critical to your success!

If you are a pear-shaped woman and have read this book from the beginning, then you're probably feeling pretty happy about your overall health situation right now. You've learned that the fat in your pear zone – including those dreaded 'saddlebags' – actually *protects* you from heart disease, type 2 diabetes and the metabolic syndrome. Your body's hormonal environment also gives you a lower risk of developing breast cancer and endometrial cancer. These are all the major killer diseases. When I look at a pear-shaped woman, I see someone who has a very good chance of living well into her 80s, 90s and beyond. Yes, you have a higher risk of osteoporosis and varicose veins than your apple-shaped sisters, but those problems are not usually life threatening. You have been blessed by your biology.

When I look at a pear-shaped woman, I see someone who has a very good chance of living well into her 80s, 90s and beyond.

Still, most pear-shaped women have a difficult time feeling grateful for the size of their thighs. I understand that, and I designed the 'Pear Shape Diet' to give you the best chance of slimming down. But my greater concern is for your overall health. Pear-shaped women are generally healthy, but if you are considerably overweight and verging on becoming an apple, with a waist-to-hip ratio (WHR) of 0.78 or higher, then I want to help you stop that progression. For near-apples I recommend using the Apple Shape Diet outlined in chapter 11. If you have a pear shape but also have high cholesterol, the metabolic syndrome or type 2 diabetes, then I also urge you to follow the Apple Shape Diet. It will help you gain control over your disease risk factors.

The Pear Shape Diet programme is designed to help pear-shaped women reduce their risk of developing osteoporosis, maintain current bone density, minimise the effects of varicose veins and reduce subcutaneous body fat. This is a much less stringent diet than the one designed for apple-shaped women because the health needs of pear-shaped women are less imminently critical. Here is what sets this diet plan apart from others:

- There is no measuring, weighing or calculating necessary.
- You won't be hungry because there are no limits on certain specified foods.
- Osteoporosis prevention is a major component.
- This programme addresses the health needs of pear-shaped women throughout their lifespan. There is no need to worry about side effects from the diet or to limit the amount of time you stay on it.

THE BODY IMAGE ISSUE

Throughout history, the pear-shaped body has been revered. Look at sculptures and paintings from just about any era and you'll see gorgeous women with rounded hips and ample thighs. Poetry, too, has idolized the pear shape. Notice the imagery in a poem titled 'The Bather', by Amy Lowell (1874–1925).

Your bright, naked body advances, blown over by leaves. . . .
Triumphant in smooth, supple roundness, edged sharp as white
*   ivory.*
Cool, perfect, with rose rarely tinting your lips and your breasts,
*   Swelling out from the green in the opulent curves of ripe fruit.*

It is the lush flesh that defines the sensuous feel of the poem. It glorifies womanly attributes, the triumph of Nature's design to match beauty with the ideal fertility form. At the time when this poem was written, and for centuries upon centuries before, curves dominated as the standard of beauty.

And then came Twiggy.

Pear-shaped women often feel like
the ugly stepsister at the fairy-tale ball.

For those of you who weren't around in the 1960s, Twiggy was an internationally famous fashion model who looked even more undernourished than Kate Moss did at her modelling peak. Thus began the trend toward the ultra-thin, angular look that continues to be popular today. It is nearly impossible for a woman to have a runway physique if she is pear-shaped. The look of the day (for the past 40-plus years) is narrow hips, a small rear end, and long, lean legs. That defines a slender apple. No wonder pear-shaped women often feel like the ugly stepsister at the fairy-tale ball.

Less Pear Than Ever

Researchers who enjoy tracking statistics have looked at the dimensions of 'ideal' women in society to see how they have changed over the years. Their published reports tell a story that pear-shaped women already know – the pear shape is no longer the most desirable. Between 1953 and 2001, the waist circumference of *Playboy* centre-folds got larger and their hip sizes got smaller. Miss America contest winners from 1921 to 1986 also had progressively larger waists. Similarly, a study that looked at British fashion models between 1967 and 1987 showed that even this elite group of women became more 'tubular', with smaller breasts and hips, and larger waists. A look at magazine images between 1970 and 1990 also discovered that the body shapes of models became less curvaceous over time, with the waist-to-hip ratio increasing significantly. This all means that the 'opulent curves of ripe fruit' are no longer valued.

There are signs that this may be changing. 'Plus-sized' models –

who start at a size 14, by the way – are becoming more popular; and a few brave pear-shaped actresses, such as Liv Tyler and Kate Winslet, are fighting the status quo by rejecting the call to become skinny-bony for the sake of their careers. (And their careers seem to be doing just fine, thank you.) Still, in most magazines and clothing catalogues, the featured models have a thin, androgynous look. I can't help but think that this aberration in aesthetics has more to do with the drape of fabric than the look of naked human beings.

Internalising the Image

Unfortunately for pear-shaped women, there are consequences from this cult of angularity. Pear-shaped women seem to have more psychological issues related to body shape, which lead them to develop eating disorders. Yale University researchers have discovered that pear-shaped women are more dissatisfied with their bodies, are less satisfied with their lives, and have lower self-esteem than apple-shaped women. It seems that lower-body fat takes on mammoth psychological significance for pear-shaped women – they are preoccupied with their hips, thighs, and buttocks to the point that their perceptions are distorted. When asked to estimate the degree to which certain body parts are overweight, pear-shaped women overshoot reality. They feel much larger than they really are. To them, their thighs are not voluptuous, they are 'thunder thighs', conjuring *Jurassic Park*–type images of women whose bodies are so large and out of control that the earth shakes when they walk. The problem is that adolescents and young women who are dissatisfied with their bodies are more likely to develop eating disorders, including anorexia and bulimia. In older women, that dissatisfaction can lead to feelings of low self-worth and depression.

An important part of health for pear-shaped women is
recognising the way society savages the body shape
that Nature intended all women to have.

I mention this here because I think that an important part of health for pear-shaped women is recognising the way society savages the body shape that Nature intended all women to have. We need to find ways to support each other in our body acceptance, and to learn to love – or at least appreciate – the pear-zone fat that will be protecting us from heart disease and type 2 diabetes. If you are like the typical pear-shaped woman, you are probably very healthy, even if you are considerably overweight. Many of the health problems caused by obesity may never apply to you because excess visceral fat is the problem, not pear-zone fat. That is a call for rejoicing. It may not feel like much of a consolation for being left out of the fashion world, but you'll be thanking your thighs when you are 70 and still active and healthy.

FAT LOSS CHALLENGES

Still, some pear-shaped women want slimmer figures. I'm sure it comes as no surprise to learn that this is easier said than done. Pear-shaped women face particular obstacles when trying to lose weight. First, pear-shaped women tend to have a lower resting metabolism than apple-shaped women. This means that, kilo for kilo, apple-shaped women burn more calories in an average day than pear-shaped women do. Apple-shaped women even burn more calories than pear-shaped women when they are sleeping. It may not be fair, but it is true. This means that a diet that works for your apple-shaped friend may not work as well or as quickly for you.

The second obstacle pear-shaped women face is that it is harder to lose pear-zone fat than it is to lose fat elsewhere in the body. If you've ever tried dieting before, then you know what happens – it seems as if you lose fat from everywhere *except* your pear zone. Your face seems to thin out, you lose fat from your breasts, and your waist even slims down. Pear-zone fat does come off, but more slowly. So after a month of dieting, you may look in the mirror and not see changes in your 'problem area'. Your trousers may not fit any more loosely – except in the waist, because any excess visceral fat you have will melt away first. This intermediate stage of dieting is dangerous for pear-shaped women because a smaller waist and shrunken breasts will create an optical illusion that their wide hips have grown even larger. This is why many pear-shaped women feel that diets and exercise don't work for them – they don't stay with the programme long enough to see the results in the pear zone. Instead, they continually seek the next great fad diet, give it 100 per cent for a few months, but then give up when they don't see the types of results they want and expect.

This type of failed expectation is the third obstacle facing pear-shaped women. Most pear-shaped women who are trying to lose weight want to lose pear-zone fat, but they don't want their breasts to shrink. Because breasts are made mostly of fat tissue, it is impossible to lose pear-zone fat without losing breast fat. (If you see a very thin actress with large breasts, chances are she has had breast augmentation surgery.) When we diet, we have an idea in mind of what we would like to look like after the diet is over. Many times, that includes losing the pear shape. For better or worse, a pear shape cannot be slimmed into a skinny apple shape. You will always have a tendency to put fat into your pear zone. You will always have wider hips than apple-shaped women. Think of it like wanting to change the length of your legs so that you become taller or shorter – it just can't happen. Even liposuction can't change a pear into an apple. Many pear-shaped women undergo this surgical procedure to have fat sucked out of their thighs with the hopes of finally having a slender lower body. Plastic surgeons know that women with large thighs who undergo liposuction are often unhappy with the results because their expectations are unreasonably high.

You are so much more than the size of your thighs. It is
time to stop playing around with fad diets, embrace
your lush, poetry-inspiring physique, and find a
programme that will help you become the healthiest
pear-shaped woman you can be.

All these shattered expectations take their toll on a pear-shaped woman's already low self-esteem. Every time a diet fails to make you toothpick thin, every time you look in a mirror and despise your buttocks, you lose a little piece of your sense of self-worth. You are so much more than the size of your thighs. It is time to stop playing around with fad diets, embrace your lush, poetry-inspiring physique and find a programme that will help you become the healthiest pear-shaped woman you can be.

In the Pear Shape Diet, I recommend a programme and specific foods that focus on the unique needs of pear-shaped women: reducing risk of osteoporosis, reducing the effects of varicose veins, minimising menopausal hot flushes and trimming pear-zone fat. These problems all have relatively straightforward solutions.

ANTI-OSTEOPOROSIS FOODS

For all the reasons described in detail in chapter 8, pear-shaped women have a higher risk of osteoporosis than apple-shaped women. It is also true that women who dieted severely before age 30, regardless of whether they were treated for an eating disorder, increase that risk. When you consider that pear-shaped women fall into eating disorders relatively easily, it's easy to see how osteoporosis is likely to plague most pear-shaped women by the time they turn 80.

Along with the hormone and pharmaceutical treatments discussed in Part 2 of this book and the exercises illustrated in chapter 13, there are several dietary steps women can take to help preserve bone density.

Calcium Supplements

Calcium is the single most important dietary factor for keeping bones strong. If we don't get enough calcium, our bodies will start to break down bone to get what they need for all the other calcium-related functions. Because of the very high risk of osteoporosis among pear-shaped women, I recommend the highest level of calcium supplements – 1,500 milligrams per day – along with a diet rich in calcium. Your body can only absorb about 500 milligrams of calcium at a time, so you'll have to take 500-milligram tablets at three separate times throughout the day.

Bone-Strengthening Foods

Even if you take calcium supplements, you'll also need to eat plenty of calcium-rich and other bone-building foods. Low-fat milk, cheese and yoghurt offer large amounts of calcium per serving. One of the best-kept calcium secrets is skimmed milk powder. Just 30g (1oz) provides 30 per cent of your calcium needs for the day. Look for ways to use powdered milk to give a calcium boost to the foods you eat daily. For example, if you mix it into your coffee instead of using liquid milk or creamer, you can get more calcium and more of that rich flavour while keeping the coffee hot. In any recipe that calls for milk, mix a little extra milk powder into the dish as well – it won't change the taste or the texture of what you are cooking. Add milk powder to your yoghurt and fruit smoothies, or sprinkle a little into your cereal. Note: many adults are lactose intolerant. Eating dairy foods will make them feel nauseated and bloated, and can cause stomach pains. If you feel bad after eating dairy foods, try getting your calcium from yoghurt (the acidophilus bacteria in yoghurt ferments the milk sugar so it won't cause digestion problems) and the other food sources listed below.

Dairy products that provide high quantities of calcium are only part of the bone-building equation – we need the balance of other minerals as well. Bones also require many other vitamins, minerals and phytochemicals to stay healthy. For example, we know that potassium, magnesium and other nutrients in fruits and vegetables are good for bones. In fact, one study showed that eating a diet high in fruits and vegetables seems to provide the ideal balance of calcium and other nutrients to protect bones. Foods that are known to contribute to bone health include potatoes, orange juice, bananas, tomatoes and tomato sauce, apples, pears (how fitting), broccoli, cauliflower, kale, pak choi, bok choy, soya foods, cantaloupe, dark breads, tea, carrots, oatmeal, fish, legumes, pasta and nuts.

You'll no doubt be thrilled to learn that a bone-healthy diet also seems to help promote weight loss. Although no one is exactly sure why, diets high in calcium – dairy foods in particular – seem to cause fat loss, *even in women who are not dieting*. Scientists suspect that calcium somehow regulates metabolism, resulting in less fat accumulation. It may also help keep metabolism burning at an optimum level. Although calcium supplements are important for preventing bone loss, they don't seem to affect weight. The loss of fat seems to come only from calcium in foods.

Avoid Sweets

On the flip side, research has shown that women who eat a lot of sweets tend to have lower bone density than women who don't eat sweets. We don't really know whether this is because the sweets displaces other, more nutritious food in the diet, or because of some chemical effect of all that sugar, but I highly recommend that pear-shaped women avoid eating sweets. Try to find a less sugar-intense way to satisfy your sweet tooth.

Calcium versus Fibre

Fibre supplements can interfere with absorption and therefore the availability of calcium in your body. If you take a fibre supplement at the same time that you take a calcium supplement, a smaller portion of the calcium will go to preserving bone density. For this reason, I don't recommend a fibre supplement for pear-shaped women. You need your calcium more than you need extra fibre. This doesn't mean that you need to avoid fibre-rich foods. On the contrary, dietary fibre is extremely important for avoiding weight gain, and for keeping your bowel movements regular – which may be quite significant for constipation-prone pear-shaped women. Eat a lot of foods that naturally contain fibre, but avoid the fibre supplements.

Soya Foods

Soyabean products are tasty, satisfying and extremely healthy for all women. Soya foods contain *phytooestrogens* – natural plant-based chemicals that work like oestrogen in the body. For pear-shaped women, this means two potential benefits: preserved bone mass density and fewer menopausal symptoms – but without the potential side effects of hormone therapy after menopause. One long-term study conducted in Japan, where women tend to eat soya foods regularly, showed that women who ate relatively high amounts of soya foods had 50 per cent fewer hot flushes than women who rarely ate soya foods.

Considering that about 85 per cent of menopausal American women experience hot flushes, adding soya foods to the diet would be a simple way to overcome those physiological 'power surges'.

Chinese researchers have discovered that women who eat soya foods often have greater bone density than women who don't eat soya foods, with the strongest effects seen five or more years after menopause. This means that after menopause, when most women are losing the largest amount of bone, women who eat soya foods are preserving more bone. What is especially important for pear-shaped women is that soya foods had the greatest effect on bone in women who had the lowest bone mass to begin with. So soya foods seem custom-designed to help pear-shaped women overcome their natural oestrogen deficit, and to add an extra measure of protection for those women who may have had an eating disorder at some time in their lives.

Soya even seems to be more effective at preserving bone than regular milk products, which also have high calcium content and have traditionally been the dietary treatment of choice for Western women trying to prevent osteoporosis. When studied side by side, both cow's milk and soya showed a general ability to help form bone. However, soya prevented more bone resorption, meaning that more of the bone-building minerals actually stayed in the bone. Milk seemed to cause more 'leakage' of calcium, with more calcium being excreted in urine. The bone-strengthening effects of soya were most pronounced among women who were not taking hormone therapy after menopause. This tells me that soya may have many of the same positive actions as oestrogen hormone therapy, without the worrisome side effects that concern some women. For example, because soya foods have no progesterone-like activity, they are unlikely to cause even the small increase in breast cancer that is seen with the typical hormone therapy. Indeed, Japanese women who eat a traditional, high-soya diet, tend to have extremely low risk of breast cancer. In addition, soya does not seem to cause any increased risk in stroke or blood clots.

These phytooestrogens are found in the highest concentrations in soya foods, but they are also found in small amounts in whole-grain cereals, flaxseed, fruits, berries and legumes. In the Pear Shape Diet, I recommend eating high quantities of all these foods.

On the other hand, I never recommend phytooestrogen supplements. These can go by many ingredient names, including 'soy protein', 'isoflavones', 'genistein', 'daidzein', or 'glycetin'. Supplements were developed to try to package the so-called active ingredient of soya foods into a megadose that can be taken by pill or powder. This is another case in which the Western culture belief that 'more is better' does not fit with the reality of medicine. Experts agree that we can only count on the positive effects of soya to come from foods, not from isolated phytooestrogens found in high amounts in supplements. Most research into these types of supplements has shown that they don't seem to work – they don't help osteoporosis, and they don't reliably prevent hot flushes. And there is a lot of concern that the pure isolates found in soya supplements may even be harmful in large doses. Instead of preventing breast cancer, soya supplements may act so similarly to oestrogen that they cause more cases of breast cancer. Scientists believe that soya foods may contain some buffering compounds that make them safe, even in large amounts – it is impossible to overdose on soya from food sources. So avoid soya protein supplements and stick with food.

These days, soya means more than just tofu. Most supermarkets carry a wide variety of soya foods that are easy to prepare and adaptable to just about anyone's taste buds. See pages 230 to 233 for more information about the types of soya-based foods available.

SALT AND SODIUM

Women who have an increased risk of varicose veins need to reduce the amount of salt in their diets. If you are pear-shaped, this means you. And if you have spider veins on your legs, your risk is higher than average – the tiniest veins in your body are already becoming varicose.

Salt increases the risk of varicose veins because it encourages water retention – and pear-shaped women tend to retain water in their legs. That fluid buildup causes additional pressure on already taxed leg veins, making it much more likely that the defective or weakened valves will fail. Tiny spider veins are the tip of the varicose iceberg.

Sodium is necessary for life, but most people get all that they need from foods that naturally contain sodium, such as meats, milk, bread and vegetables. Any more than the bare minimum just goes to increase fluid retention and cause high blood pressure. It is in every pear-shaped woman's interest to severely restrict dietary salt to avoid the leg pain, fatigue and swelling that accompany enlarged veins. Added dietary salt can become almost addictive because it deadens your taste buds. The more salt you eat, the more you'll need in order to derive any taste from your food. Plus, evidence suggests that we become less sensitive to salt as we get older, so if you are eating large amounts of salt now, you'll need even more to get the same taste in a few years. It becomes a vicious cycle of needing more and more salt to continue to enjoy food, which means more and more water retention, more weight gain and more leg discomfort.

Unfortunately, there is no way to shake the salt habit except to go cold turkey. It will be unpleasant for three weeks, and you may even get irritable during that time as your body chemistry readjusts and you are forced to deal with flavourless meals. Simply cutting down on salt (instead of cutting out salt entirely) will be unsatisfying to you and will still be dampening your taste, so it will feel like extended torture. On the other hand, if you stop eating salt right now, all food will taste bland only for about ten days to three weeks – the amount of time it takes for new receptor cells to develop in the taste buds. After that, foods you thought tasted just fine before will now be too salty. Not only that, but you may develop a much finer sense of taste overall. Studies show that taste receptors can change, so that a 'salt' taste receptor can turn into a 'sweet' taste receptor. By laying off the salt, you will become more sensitive to salt, but you may also find that other tastes become more intense as well. And you'll be making yourself healthier at the same time.

Your goal, then, is to cut as much salt out of your diet as possible. At a very basic level, this means never adding salt to food at the table. Throw the saltshaker in the same closet you threw your bathroom scales – don't keep it around. Other salt-reducing tips:

◆ Use only small amounts of salt when you are cooking, and add it early in the cooking process to enhance the natural flavours of foods.

◆ Read food labels. Next to table salt, added salt in processed foods is the greatest source of sodium in our diets. Look for 'low sodium' or 'no sodium' labels on frozen and canned foods.

◆ Use herbs for flavour instead of salt. If you can handle spicy tastes, try adding chilli pepper or curry powder. Basil, garlic, lemon, oregano, rosemary, mint and thyme will add new dimensions to the taste of foods – experiment with them to discover which you prefer in your cooking.

◆ Avoid foods that are prepared with large amounts of salt, especially deli meats (look for low-sodium varieties), pickles, anchovies, salted nuts, olives, potato crisps, pretzels, crackers, soya sauce and broth or bullion cubes – if it tastes salty, then you can be sure it contains too much salt.

◆ Unless you sweat a lot during strenuous exercise, avoid sports drinks, such as Lucozade. These drinks were originally designed for athletes who lose a great amount of sodium when they sweat. Now, many nonathletes drink sports drinks, but they are not a healthy drink for relatively sedentary people. They contain sodium and quite a bit of sugar – sodium will contribute to water retention, and sugar will contribute to accumulated fat.

FAT, FAT AND FAT

One hypothesis for why pear-shaped women have a lower risk of type 2 diabetes and heart disease is that visceral fat cells are inherently different from pear-zone fat cells. Visceral fat cells – the kind that apple-shaped women have trouble with – have poor insulin sensitivity. After a fatty meal, the fatty acids produced in visceral fat escape into the bloodstream, where they can do their disease damage. On the other hand, pear-zone fat cells have good insulin sensitivity. After a fatty meal, pear-zone fat will suck up the fatty acids and store them immediately – and they are *stored as fat in the pear zone*. So while this storage of fatty acids helps protect pear-shaped women from disease, it is also a wonderfully efficient system for the growth and maintenance of rounded hips, thighs and buttocks.

Low-Fat Diets Help Pear-Shaped Women

One logical fix is to eat a diet very low in fat. In fact, researchers believe that low-fat eating is crucial for weight loss and weight maintenance in pear-shaped women. Once you lose weight from your pear zone, the fat cells are still there – they decrease in size, but not in number – so you will still have disease protection. And if you maintain a low-fat diet, you should also be able to keep from filling those fat cells back up again. One very pear-shaped woman I know (with a WHR of 0.66) swears by what she calls a No Cheese Diet whenever she wants to lose weight. All she does is stop eating cheese and other blatantly fatty foods for three months and she drops a full trouser size. Given the metabolic actions of pear-zone fat, this makes perfect sense. A study published in 2004 found that eating a high-carbohydrate, low-fat diet helps women significantly decrease their thigh fat in just 12 weeks. Yes, that's right – *thigh* fat. And the weight loss was accomplished without decreasing metabolism. The carbohydrates recommended were the 'complex' carbohydrates – those with a lot of fibre and a minimum of sugar and fats. The Pear Shape Diet recommends these kinds of high-quality carbohydrates as the main portion of your diet.

Eating a high-carbohydrate, low-fat diet can help women decrease their thigh fat.

Types of Fats Make a Difference

Even changing the type of fat eaten may help women slim. There are three main types of fats: saturated fats, monounsaturated fats and polyunsaturated fats. The word 'saturated' pertains to chemical structure, not to any action on the body or food content.

Saturated fats are fats that are solid at room temperature. These are fats from animal products, such as the fat in full cream milk, cheese, butter, ice cream, lard and the solid fat found in meats. Palm oil and coconut oil – sometimes called 'tropical oils' on food labels – are also saturated fats. When women stop eating saturated fats and replace them with mono- or polyunsaturated fats, they lose subcutaneous fat – the kind pear-shaped women have the most.

Monounsaturated fats, found primarily in olive oil and rapeseed oil, are among the healthiest fats. Therefore, these are the only oils I recommend for cooking at home.

Polyunsaturated fats are divided into three categories:

1. Omega-3 fatty acids, the most beneficial of the fats, are found in many kinds of fish, shellfish, rapeseed oil, soyabeans, wheatgerm, flaxseed and walnuts.

2. Omega-6 fatty acids are also necessary for good health, but we don't have to seek them out. They are plentiful in many of the foods

we eat, including meats, corn oil, safflower oil, 'vegetable' oils, leafy vegetables, seeds, nuts and grains.

3. *Trans*-fatty acids are a man-made invention and are unhealthy for everybody. By taking a polyunsaturated oil and changing the chemical structure, scientists were able to solidify the oil so it could be used for baking and in butter-substitute margarine spreads. The different chemical structure also gives the fat a longer shelf life. Butter and oils go rancid pretty quickly, but trans fats can stay around almost forever. The problem is that by changing the chemical structure, these fats were made more dangerous than saturated fats, and it is very possible that they are a major contributor to your pear-zone fat. If you read the ingredient lists on food labels, the words 'partially hydrogenated' mean that oil was turned into a trans fat. Put the product back on the shelf. Consumers have become savvy about shopping for products that don't contain trans fats, and manufacturers have responded. Look for labels that say 'No Trans Fats' on bread, biscuits or other baked goods.

No one can eat a totally fat-free diet because many foods naturally contain fat, and you wouldn't want to – fats are important for building cell membranes and manufacturing some hormones. But pear-shaped women who are concerned with their weight will lose fat more quickly and more successfully if they eat a diet very low in fat – let's call it 'excess-fat free'.

Not only will less fat help reduce the size of your thighs, but it may also help preserve your bones. Researchers in the United Kingdom tracked the eating habits and bone mass density of nearly 900 middle-aged women for five to seven years. They discovered that women who ate higher amounts of even the 'good' fats – the monounsaturated and polyunsaturated fats – lost significantly more bone than women who ate less fats. So eating low-fat helps pear-shaped women lose pear-zone fat and preserve bone strength.

Eating low-fat helps pear-shaped women lose pear-zone fat and preserve bone strength.

Encouragement for Low-Fat Eating

Many women hear the words 'low fat' and immediately stop listening. They think that low fat is the same as low flavour. It's easy to understand why. Eating fat is hardwired into our bodies to be enjoyable. Fat, with its high calorie count and easy storage, enabled our primitive ancestors to survive times of famine. It's part of our genetics to enjoy eating fatty foods. However, part of our enjoyment comes from pure habit. When we eat fatty foods, our bodies produce enzymes, called 'lipase', to break down the fats. When we eat a meal, the body releases lipase to help digest the fat and allow it to be used by the body. Because most of us have a pretty consistent diet, our bodies learn approximately how much lipase will be needed, and that is the amount that is produced.

So let's say you are a woman who eats very little fat most of the time. Your body will produce very small amounts of lipase. If you eat a very fatty meal for a change, you will feel sick – the body doesn't have enough lipase ready to handle the extra fat load, so there is no immediate way to break down the fats. Instead of being digested, the fats just slither through the gastrointestinal tract. Chances are you will later have a bout of diarrhoea as the fat makes its way relatively intact to your bowel. So even though our taste for fatty foods is partly genetic, our individual habits can break that need for fat. After enough time on a low-fat diet, eating fatty foods will no longer be enjoyable – they will make you nauseous instead. My overall message is that you have to be patient with a low-fat diet. You have to give your body time to adjust. After a few months, you won't even want those foods you crave most now.

Calories

The trick with low-fat diets, as we've learned in the past 10 years, is that you can't substitute high-calorie foods for your high-fat favourites and still accomplish your health goals. The point is to eat better quality foods, not poor-quality foods with the fat taken out. If you eat a box of biscuits, whether they are high-fat or low-fat, you will gain weight. If you are on a diet to lose weight or get healthy, you have to stop looking for the loopholes. Nature isn't fooled by a list of ingredients on a box. Naturally occurring low-fat foods – not the kind constructed in a laboratory – are almost always low-calorie foods. Fats contain more calories per gram than carbohydrates and proteins. A gram of either a carbohydrate or a protein contains 4 calories; but a gram of fat contains 9 calories – more than double. It would make logical sense to think that if you take the fat out of a biscuit, it should be much lower in calories. Unfortunately, that's not the way it works. If you just take the fat out of a biscuit, it would taste pretty awful, so manufacturers add in lots of sugars to compensate. The result is a biscuit with little fat but more sugar than the typical biscuit, so you really don't lose many calories. As I explained in chapter 10, calories are a critical component of weight loss. If we eat more calories than we burn off, we will gain weight. That's the catch with artificially low-fat foods – they tend to either taste bad or have additional sugar calories. Naturally low-fat foods, on the other hand, are low in calories and taste good – the way Nature intended.

You have to stop looking for the loopholes. Nature isn't fooled by a list of ingredients on a box.

In the Pear Shape Diet, I recommend avoiding artificially low-fat foods as much as possible. If the choice comes down to a full-fat biscuit and a low-fat biscuit (and you won't be talked out of it) I would rather have you eat the full-fat biscuit and be satisfied, than to have you eat a box of low-fat biscuits and still feel cheated.

THE PEAR SHAPE DIET PROGRAMME

Important note: apple-shaped people — men, women or children — should not follow this diet. Low fat is not a good choice for them — they need moderate amounts of fat for optimal weight loss and to keep their levels of healthy HDL cholesterol from dropping. If you have an apple-shaped family member, many of the recommended foods are in both plans, so you can make compatible meals.

Now that you understand the principles behind the recommendations, the basics of the Pear Shape Diet are simple.

1. *You can eat as many 'Slim' foods as you want.* Slim foods are naturally low in fat and low in sodium, and many are high in calcium. For any meal, for any snack, if you eat *Slim* foods then you don't have to weigh, measure or count anything. Of course, use common sense about portions. This is not a prescription for gorging yourself, even if the foods are healthy. It's just that you don't have to measure out half a cup of brown rice or count out twelve grapes. Simply eat a satisfying amount. Too much of anything will cause you to gain weight.

2. To lose girth faster, keep applying the 25 per cent solution. I would rather have you stick to the diet than to cut calories in the beginning, but if you can do both, you'll lose more weight more quickly.

3. Begin eliminating all extraneous fats from your diet. This means the butter or margarine on your toast, the cheese in your salad and

the oil or mayonnaise on your sandwich. Many foods have fats in them, so try not to add more fats on top of the food. To avoid cravings, start by using only half the amount you do now. After a week, reduce that by half again. In another week, cut the amount again. Keep reducing your fat use until you have kicked the fat habit.

4. Hide the saltshaker and vow never to add salt at the table again. At the same time, cut the amount of salt you use in cooking by half. Look for low-sodium packaged foods.

5. Add calcium-rich foods to your diet. Aim to eat at least one 'High Calcium' food at each meal, for a total of a minimum of three High Calcium foods per day. Many of these foods are also on the Slim foods list, so don't be surprised if you see them twice.

6. Add soya foods to your diet. If you don't already eat soya foods, aim to eat three soya foods per week. Work your way up to eating soya foods a *minimum* of six times per week.

7. Avoid all 'Zoned-Out' foods. These are fatty, salty or osteoporosis-causing foods – all the foods that keep your pear zone filled out and that increase your risks for the disorders that haunt pear-shaped women. If you cannot avoid them entirely, cut down as much as possible. If you do eat Zoned-Out foods, limit the damage by applying the 25 per cent solution.

8. Foods from the 'Moderate' list are not as healthy as foods in the Slim list, but they are also not as unhealthy as foods in the Zoned-Out list. They should be eaten infrequently. Always apply the 25 per cent solution to Moderate foods. Aim to eat no more than five Moderate foods per day.

9. Eat three meals and three snacks each day. It is OK to skip a snack, but it is never OK to skip a meal – it just sets you up for overeating later in the day.

High Calcium Foods

The foods listed here contain relatively high amounts of calcium. I am not including the actual milligram counts because I don't want you to bother with that – my goal is to get you to stop weighing yourself down with numbers. Ideally you should try to eat at least one High Calcium food at each meal. Eat a variety of foods from this list to increase your odds of getting all the nutrients necessary for strong bones. After a while, eating foods from this list will seem like second nature.

High Calcium Choices

Skimmed milk	*Broccoli*	*Turnip greens*
Low-fat yoghurt	*Brussels sprouts*	*Watercress*
Low-fat cottage cheese	*Cauliflower*	*Rhubarb*
Tofu	*Spring greens*	*Watermelon*
Fortified soya milk	*French beans*	*Oranges*
Lentils	*Runner beans*	*Figs*
Pinto beans	*Kale*	*Molasses*
Chickpeas	*Sweet potatoes*	
Pak choi (a leafy green)	*Swiss chard*	

Breakfast

◆ **Eat breakfast every day.** Studies have shown that people who eat breakfast are about half as likely to be obese as people who don't eat breakfast. The myth is that if you only eat two meals a day, you're cutting out one-third of your daily calories, so you'll have to lose weight. Not true. Most people make up for morning hunger by eating more – and more Zoned-Out foods – later in the day.

Note: The choices in the following charts are suggestions based on typical foods eaten at these particular meals. There is no reason why you could not eat pasta for breakfast, or a low-fat muesli for dinner. Feel free to mix and match Slim foods whenever you feel like eating them.

Breakfast Choices

ZONED-OUT	MODERATE	SLIM
Most American-style muffins	Fortified soya milk	Whole fruit – any kind
Cinnamon rolls	Semi-skimmed milk	Wholemeal bread
Croissants	Bagels, plain	Multigrain bread
Brioches	Meat substitutes	Rye bread
Danish pastry	Sausages (soya)	Pumpernickel bread
Doughnuts	Bacon (soya)	Low-fat cottage cheese
Scones	Whole eggs	Low-fat yoghurt
Sugary breakfast cereal	White bread	Porridge
Fatty breakfast cereal*	Nuts/peanut butter	Breakfast cereals
Fried potatoes	Most pancakes	Whole-grain
Any kind of sausage	Muffins	Fat-free muesli
Bacon	Low-fat cheese	Egg whites
Cheese		Wholewheat pancakes
Butter		Dried fruits
Margarine		Applesauce
Olive and other oils		Fruit juice
Full cream milk		Coffee
Cream		Tea
*A 'fatty' breakfast cereal is one that contains more than three grams of fat per 100g (3½oz) of cereal. This information can be found on the ingredients label.		Green tea
		Skimmed milk
		Jam or marmalade
		Honey
		(virtually) Non fat cream cheese

Suggestions ...

◆ Wholemeal or multigrain toast with jam, marmalade or honey.

◆ A plain bagel with virtually no-fat cream cheese; if desired, add pineapple chunks.

◆ Low-fat whole-grain cereal or fat-free muesli with skimmed milk. Add berries or bananas.

◆ Soya milk (vanilla) or skimmed milk smoothie, made by blending your choice of milk with your choice of fruit. My favourite is half a banana with a cup of blueberries, strawberries, or raspberries.

◆ Cottage cheese or yoghurt with fruit and a touch of honey.

◆ Scrambled egg whites with a little soft tofu mixed in for texture. Serve on a muffin with a slice of tomato.

◆ If you make American-style muffins at home using a fat substitute, they can become a Slim food. Good substitutes are applesauce, prune purée or pumpkin purée. If the recipe calls for butter, use half a cup of applesauce instead. I do not recommend store-bought baked goods, even if they are fat-free, because they are apt to contain much higher amounts of sugar. If you substitute molasses for sugar, you'll have a High Calcium food, too.

◆ Remember not to spread butter or margarine on baked goods.

◆ Feel free to drink coffee or tea – just don't add cream, full-cream milk or low-fat milk. Try fortified soya milk instead, or skimmed milk with added nonfat dry milk.

◆ **Take a multivitamin with breakfast.** No one eats a perfectly balanced diet all the time. In order to catch all the necessary nutrients, I recommend taking a multivitamin every day. The vitamin you choose should supply 400 micrograms of folic acid (folate), 400 IU vitamin D, 6 micrograms vitamin B_{12}, and 3 milligrams vitamin B$_6$. Premenopausal women also need 15 milligrams of iron. After menopause, taking additional iron in a supplement may actually contribute to heart disease. My personal favourite multivitamins for premenopausal women are regular Centrum. For postmenopausal women I recommend Centrum Select 50+. Some people just have a hard time swallowing pills. For them, I recommend looking for chewable children's vitamins. Believe it or not, chewing just one is great for premenopausal women. Postmenopausal women can chew tablets which do not contain iron.

◆ **Take one 500-milligram calcium supplement at each meal.** The form of calcium in most supplements is calcium carbonate, which can cause constipation in some women. Because pear-shaped women suffer from constipation more often than apple-shaped women, I recommend that pear-shaped women take a supplement that contains calcium citrate, which does not cause constipation. If you don't have constipation problems, you might want to try chewable Ellactiva calcium supplements. They make remembering to take your vitamins a joy – and because sweets are on the *Zoned-Out* list for pear-shaped women, here's your chance to get a guilt-free treat three times a day.

Midmorning

◆ **Eat a midmorning snack if you are hungry.**

◆ **Always carry a Slim snack in your handbag or briefcase.** If you are not prepared, you may be tempted to buy vending machine food, all of which is to be avoided. But if you have a snack plan, you'll be less likely to be seduced by unhealthy food in a moment of weakness.

Snack Choices

ZONED-OUT	MODERATE	SLIM
Sweets	Frozen yoghurt	Whole fruit – any kind
Sweet biscuits/cookies	Low-fat cheese	Vegetables
Most American-style muffins	No-salt fat-free popcorn	Wholemeal bread
Cinnamon rolls	No-salt pretzels	Multigrain bread
Croissants	Soya milk	Pumpernickel bread
Danish pastry	Regular yoghurt	Rye bread
Doughnuts	Plain digestive bisuits	Dried fruits
Scones		Fat-free muesli bar
Cheese		Low-fat cereal
Crackers		Low-fat yoghurt
Popcorn, with butter and salt		Low-fat cottage cheese
French fries		Coffee
Potato crisps		Tea
Corn chips		Green tea
Pretzels, regular		Skimmed milk
Ice cream		Fruit juice
Cream dressings		(virtually) No-fat cream cheese
Full cream milk		(virtually) No-fat fromage frais
Cream		Ice lolly
Cola drinks		
Sports drinks		
'Diet' drinks		

Suggestions . . .

◆ Dried fruit can taste like sweets, and it contains concentrated amounts of nutrients. Experiment with different varieties. Many supermarkets and health food stores have large selections, including bananas, pineapples, apples, mangos, apricots, papayas, pears, cherries, cranberries, prunes and raisins.

◆ Sliced or baby carrots, celery stalks, red pepper wedges, cucumber slices, courgette sticks or broccoli florets with a fat-free yoghurt or tofu dressing dip.

◆ Sprinkle low-fat cereal into a cup of low-fat yoghurt. Add honey or jam for a sweeter treat.

◆ Fruit salad, alone or with low-fat yoghurt or low-fat cottage cheese. Whole fresh fruit is best, frozen fruit is next best. If you are really in a time pinch, you can use tinned fruit salad.

◆ Make your own snack mix of dried fruits, soya nuts (like peanuts, but made from soya beans) and low-fat muesli. I make a snack mix and place it in a sandwich for airline travel or a quick snack if I'm on the road. My favourite mixture is no-salt soya nuts, sunflower seeds, dried cranberries, pumpkin seeds and cashew pieces.

Lunch

◆ **Don't forget to take your second calcium supplement.**

◆ **Prepare your own lunch so that you can control the ingredients.** Eating out for lunch is a trial when you are trying to eat healthily. The world conspires to make you choose *Zoned-Out* foods. If you bring your own lunch to work or have something handy at home, you'll be less tempted to eat fatty or salty foods.

Lunch Choices

ZONED-OUT	MODERATE	SLIM
Anything fried	White bread	Whole fruit – any kind
Anything made with trans fats	Bread sticks	Vegetables
	Crusty rolls	Salad
Cheese	French bread	Wholemeal bread
Crackers/savoury biscuits	Soya products	Pumpernickel bread
	Veggie burgers	Rye bread
Cheese rolls	Veggie hot dogs	Multigrain bread
Beef	Ham	Legumes, lentils
Hot dogs	Low-fat cheese	Pasta
Hamburger	Chicken	Wholewheat pasta
Fried chicken	Turkey	Tagliatelle verdi
Polish sausage	Fish*	Tortillas, any type
Salami	Nuts, peanut butter	Tomato sauce
Pastrami	Semi-skimmed milk	Low-fat cottage cheese
Bologna	Soya milk	Low-fat yoghurt
Corned beef		Coffee
Chorizo	*Tuna, swordfish, shark and	Tea
Spareribs	marlin are not Elite because	Green tea
Bacon	they tend to contain high	Fruit juice
Corn chips, regular	levels of mercury, which can	Skimmed milk
Pretzels, regular	be harmful if eaten in large	Low-fat mayonnaise
Ice cream	quantities. Women who are	No-fat dressing
Cream dressings	pregnant, breastfeeding or	(virtually) No-fat
Full cream milk	trying to conceive should eat	fromage frais
Cream	no more than two medium-	Ice lolly
Sweets	sized tins of tuna, or one tuna	Dried fruit
Cola drinks	steak, per week. Pregnant	Fresh lemonade
Energy drinks	women, infants and children	
'Diet' drinks	under 16 years of age should	
	avoid eating shark, swordfish	
	and marlin.	

Suggestions . . .

◆ Make your own cheese-free pizza with tomato sauce, tofu and your favourite green vegetable.

◆ Bake a whole potato the night before. When it has cooled, cut the potato in half lengthwise and scoop out some (not all) of the flesh. Load the inside of the potato 'boats' with diced tomatoes, kidney beans and some spinach leaves. For lunch, heat the potato boats in a microwave and serve with a fat-free soured cream.

◆ Experiment with fat-free dressings or sauces to use as bread toppings.

◆ If you buy cold meats, look for low-sodium, low-fat varieties.

Afternoon Snack

◆ **Eat an afternoon snack if you are hungry.** This snack is what I called the 'excuse snack'. We may not be hungry, but it's a great excuse to take a break from work, or sit down with the kids after school, or procrastinate before making dinner or starting some other evening project. Resolve to make this snack as healthy as possible so that you know you are eating from hunger and not from boredom or another excuse. If you are not hungry enough to eat something healthy, then maybe you don't need the snack. Use the same snack list as for the midmorning snack.

Dinner

◆ **Don't forget to take your third calcium supplement.**

Dinner Choices

ZONED-OUT	MODERATE	SLIM
Anything fried	White bread	Whole fruit – any kind
Anything made with trans fats	French bread	Vegetables, not fried
Olives	Crusty rolls	Potatoes
Pickles	Bread sticks	Root vegetables
Cheese	White rice	Legumes, lentils
Cheese rolls	Ham	Salad
Crackers	Pork shoulder	Wholemeal bread
Savoury biscuits	Pork chops	Multigrain bread
Pork chops	Roast pork leg	Pumpernickel bread
Hot dogs	Chicken	Rye bread
Hamburger	Turkey	Pitta
Fried chicken	Fish	Tortillas, any kind
Polish sausage	Venison	Tempeh
Salami	Oysters, clams	Tofu
Pastrami	Mussels	Pasta
Bologna	Soya products	Wholewheat pasta
Corned beef	Veggie burgers	Tagliatelle verdi
Chorizo	Veggie hot dogs	Brown rice*
Spareribs	Meat substitutes	Bulgar wheat*
Bacon	Nuts	Wheat berries*
Spam	Hummus	Quinoa*
Duck	Polenta	Couscous
Goose	Semi-skimmed milk	Tomato sauce
Panfried pork chops		(virtually) No-fat dressings
Lamb		(virtually) No-fat cream cheese
Veal		
Cream dressings		*Box in chapter 11 (page 248–249) describes how to cook these grains.
Full cream milk		

Suggestions...

◆ Use dried and fresh fruits in your meals to add flavour and texture to a meal. For example, pineapple and mango complement many meat dishes; and finely diced dried apples, prunes, dried apricots or raisins make a tasty addition to rice or other grains.

◆ Become creative with tortillas. The popular wrap sandwich concept can extend to dinner. Create a veggie wrap using your favourite combination of ingredients, then slice the wrap crosswise into one-inch pieces so that you get little rounds with a swirl in the middle. Serve with your choice of toppings, such as low-fat soured cream, salsa, fat-free dressing or tomato sauce. I like to make wraps the day before, then reheat them in the microwave for a quick dinner.

◆ 'Kitchen Sink Risotto' – a great way to use leftover cooked vegetables. In a large pot, bring 1.4 litres (2½ pints) of chicken or vegetable broth to a boil, then let simmer. Meanwhile, dice one small onion and three cloves of garlic. Sauté them in two tablespoons of oil in a large frying pan over medium heat. When the onions are clear but not brown, add 340ml (12fl oz) of Arborio rice (sometimes called risotto rice). This type of rice absorbs much more liquid than long-grain white rice, creating a creamy-tasting dish with very little fat. Stir until the grains of rice are coated with oil, about one minute. Stir in 115ml (4fl oz) of white wine. When it has been absorbed, add 115ml (4fl oz) of the simmering broth. Stir constantly, adding 115ml (4fl oz) broth whenever the added liquid has been mostly absorbed. When you have used about half of the broth, stir in any combination of cooked vegetables you want, or that you have left over. I enjoy asparagus and chives; artichokes and sun-dried tomatoes; dried mushrooms; and sweetcorn, beans and tomatoes. Continue adding the liquid as before until all the broth has been absorbed, or until the rice is tender. The cooking process usually takes about 20 minutes.

Desserts

As a physician, I am not in favour of anyone eating dessert (except fruit, of course). However, as a human being, I know that I can't always resist sweet foods. My recommendation is to eat desserts only on the weekends. If you currently eat something sweet every day, the weekend dessert plan will cut your sweets consumption by about two-thirds. Whenever possible, try to eat Slim desserts. They will satisfy your sweet tooth without fat.

You can make many desserts on the Zoned-Out list healthier by making them at home, replacing fats with applesauce or prune purée. Always avoid sweets because of their contribution to osteoporosis.

Dessert Choices

ZONED-OUT	MODERATE	SLIM
Sweets	Nuts	Whole fruit – any kind
Most gateaux and cakes	Soya-milk smoothie	Applesauce
American-style muffins	Homemade cake	Sorbet
Cinnamon rolls		Ice lolly
Cookies		Frozen low-fat yoghurt
Danish pastry		Ice milk
Doughnuts		Hard muesli bars
Ice cream		Dried fruits
Chocolate		Skimmed-milk pudding

Evening Snack

◆ **Eat an evening snack if you need to.** This is the most optional of all the snacks. My usual recommendation is not to eat anything after 8 P.M., but I understand that this habit can be difficult to break. Try not to go into the kitchen after dinner. If you must have a snack, use the same list as for the midmorning snack.

CHAPTER 13

Apples and Pears Exercise Programme

I f I had a magic genie that could grant me one wish that would do the greatest good for the most people, it would be that people would learn to find joy in physical activity. Exercise is the single most powerful weapon we have in our personal health arsenal. You want to fight heart disease? Exercise is the best way to do it. Type 2 diabetes? Exercise. Depression, obesity, fatigue, osteoporosis, stress? Exercise, exercise, exercise. I'm not telling you anything you haven't heard hundreds of times before. For those of you who hate the very word 'exercise', call it whatever you want – physical activity, fitness, working out or training – you and I both know that you need to *move*.

If I had a magic genie that could grant me one wish
that would do the greatest good for the most people,
it would be that people would learn to find joy in
physical activity.

And yet, 70 per cent of women don't get nearly enough exercise to stay healthy. A full 25 per cent of us admit that we are totally sedentary, getting no exercise at all. Why? Many physicians believe it is because people are just too lazy to get up off the couch. I don't believe that's true. When I ask my patients, they tell me exactly why they don't exercise, and never has 'laziness' been one of the reasons. Read through this top 10 list of reasons and put a check mark next to the ones that are true for you.

❏ **No time.** Your days are packed with other responsibilities from morning until bedtime.

❏ **Hate exercising.** You can't stand the whole process, and you don't find it enjoyable.

❏ **It hurts.** You find it painful to exercise, either immediately or the next day.

❏ **Forgetfulness or different priorities.** You want to exercise, you have every intention of exercising, but you either forget or get distracted by some other activity.

❏ **No equipment.** You have no space to store a treadmill or other piece of equipment, or you don't have the extra money to spend on that type of luxury item.

❏ **It's just a fad.** Running, jogging, walking . . . tai chi, yoga, Pilates . . . aerobics, stair-stepping, spinning. It's like trying to keep up with the latest fashion – but just when you've got the hang of one exercise, something new comes along.

❏ **Low return on your time investment.** You tried exercising before, but it didn't seem to do you any good. Why bother doing something if you can't see the results?

❏ **Not safe.** You live in a neighbourhood where it is dangerous to walk, either because of traffic or crime.

❏ **No one ever told you why exercise is important.** Sure,

the doctor told you to exercise, but you don't know exactly what the specific benefits are.

❏ **Confusion or frustration.** You don't know exactly which exercises to do, or it all seems too complicated.

None of those sound like laziness to me, so let's start breaking down the barriers.

WHY EXERCISE IS IMPORTANT

Exercise does more than just strengthen our muscles and burn calories. As I've discussed throughout this book, our bodies are amazing biological communities where every cell has a job to do, communication among body parts occurs at the speed of a thought and all our tissues work together to keep us alive and functioning. When we exercise, our hearts pump faster so that blood circulates more efficiently. Body temperature rises, metabolism gets fired up, certain hormone levels rise or fall, endorphins – the body's natural painkillers – are released, and hundreds of other physiologic changes occur.

Women who walk at a moderately brisk pace just 30 minutes a day, every day, have improved insulin sensitivity, reduced levels of dangerous LDL cholesterol, lower blood pressure, and healthier blood vessels. This relatively small amount of exercise can help reduce their risk of heart disease, stroke, and type 2 diabetes by about 30 per cent. Women who exercise regularly also experience less depression and anxiety, and have fewer and milder premenstrual and menopausal symptoms.

Over the long term, exercise can help prevent colon cancer, breast cancer, lung cancer, osteoporosis, osteoarthritis and even dementia. One long-term study tested cardiovascular fitness and cognitive function at the beginning of the study and again six years later. The researchers discovered that the participants who had the worst fitness level at the beginning of the study also had the worst scores on thinking ability six years later. The participants who had good fitness levels at the beginning of the study performed the best six years later, with no decline in mental abilities. This makes sense when you consider that exercise helps keep arteries clear – including arteries in the brain. If you have good blood flow to the brain, your mind will stay sharp.

A little physical activity can also reduce inflammation in the body with an effect similar to taking corticosteroid medications. This equates to less risk of disease, as well as reduced pain from arthritis and other inflammation-related disorders. And if you're not yet convinced that exercise is the active equivalent of a wonder drug, here's an added bonus: twenty minutes of intense exercise – regardless of your overall level of fitness – has been shown to increase a woman's physical response to sexual arousal.

The benefits of physical activity are global – they are not confined to the particular area of the body that is being exercised. Walking does more than strengthen your legs (although it does that very effectively). Walking also helps change your overall body chemistry to make you healthier from head to toe. *That* is why exercise is so important. It's not about your thighs or your stomach or any other single body part – it is about your entire body.

Fitness Is More Important Than Fat

One of the most exciting and heartening research results of the past few years has to be the acknowledgment that a woman can be fit even if she is overweight, with all the same health benefits that come from being lean and fit. This is a more inclusive view of what 'physical fitness' means, concentrating on the health of the body instead of on weight alone. In fact, studies have shown that people who are overweight and physically fit have a lower risk of heart attack and type

2 diabetes than those who are of normal weight but not physically fit. This tells us that it is better to be fit and fat than to be thin and not fit. Exercise confers health, even if body mass index remains relatively high.

People who are overweight and physically fit have a
lower risk of heart attack and type 2 diabetes than
those who are of normal weight but not physically fit.

Research also tells us that it's never too late to reap the health benefits of exercise. One fascinating study followed the exercise habits and health of a group of over 7,500 women for about six years. Based on the women's own reports, they were divided into four groups for comparison: (1) women who were active and remained active throughout the study; (2) women who were sedentary and remained sedentary throughout the study; (3) women who were active but became sedentary; and (4) women who were sedentary but became active. As expected, women who had always been active had about a 40 per cent lower risk of death from heart disease or cancer than women who had always been sedentary. What was really amazing, however, was that the group of women who had been sedentary but became active ended up with about the same disease risk levels as women who had always been active. Right from the first year of follow-up, women who started a new exercise programme had the same low risk of disease as women who had been exercising for years. By the end of the study, these newly active women lowered their overall risk of death by 36 per cent. Please don't use this information as an excuse to delay starting to exercise – there are other health benefits that accrue along the way. But I find this information inspiring, and a confirmation of the resilience of the human body. The take-home message is that even if you have never exercised, starting a fitness programme will benefit you immediately.

Imagine a 36 per cent lower risk of death just by taking a daily walk. It is a breathtakingly potent activity.

Even if you have never exercised, starting a fitness program will benefit you immediately. Imagine a 36 per cent lower risk of death just by taking a daily walk. It is a breathtakingly potent activity.

EXERCISE FOR LOSING FAT

Of course, fat loss is the main reason why most women exercise. The bottom line is that it really does work. Physical activity alone has been shown to reduce visceral fat and total body fat – including pear-zone fat – in all women, regardless of whether they are of normal weight or overweight. And overweight women with a family history of obesity lose proportionately more fat than women without such an inheritance. This means that regardless of how overweight you are now or how much your body naturally tends towards fatness, you can make it slimmer through physical activity.

Regardless of how overweight you are now or how much your body naturally tends toward fatness, you can make it slimmer through physical activity.

Exercise is more effective than dieting at helping women lose weight and keep weight off. Dieting lowers metabolism, which means that weight will eventually creep back on, even if you keep dieting. Exercise helps maintain the lean body tissue that revs up metabolism, so you'll lose weight without the same diet-induced metabolism problem. This means that the weight will stay off longer.

Some studies have shown that visceral fat tends to be lost first, so apple-shaped women may meet their fat-loss targets faster than pear-shaped women. One study looked at what happened to visceral fat stores in postmenopausal women who walked about 25 minutes per day, about four days per week. After 12 months, the women didn't lose very much actual body weight, but they lost a considerable amount of visceral fat. This is one of the reasons that I recommend throwing away the bathroom scales. Weight isn't your best measure of health, or even of how well a diet or exercise programme is working. These women lost significant amounts of fat from around their waists – reducing their risks of heart disease and diabetes – but none of that was reflected on the scales. I have heard this from many of my patients. One pear-shaped woman told me that she exercised by walking daily, went down two dress sizes, but never lost a pound. She said that she feels more compact, almost as if she is wearing a girdle. When we add muscle and lose fat, we may not lose weight, but we'll look and feel better – and be all-around healthier.

Of course, coupling moderate exercise with a moderate diet is the best option of all. In a 16-month study, women who exercised and dieted reduced their visceral fat stores by 5 per cent; women who only exercised stayed the same weight; and women who neither exercised nor dieted *gained* an additional 5 per cent of fat in their abdomen. In these days of growing obesity, maintaining weight can be considered a victory for many women, so exercise alone is helpful. But exercise plus diet will slim your silhouette. It is estimated that combining diet with exercise helps women lose about five times as much visceral fat as dieting alone. Those dramatic results are good news to apple-shaped women who are looking for an effective way to trim their waists.

Combining diet with exercise helps women lose about
five times as much visceral fat as dieting alone.

TYPES OF EXERCISE

There are two main types of exercise: *aerobic* and *anaerobic*. The word
'aerobic' means *requiring oxygen*. Simply speaking, aerobic exercises are
those that can make you feel out of breath because the body's oxygen
needs are so high. These include walking, jogging, running, swimming,
cycling and anything else that makes your heart pump and causes you
to breathe heavily after a while. Aerobic exercises are intended to be
done at relatively low intensity, but for a rather long time – 30 to 60
minutes or longer. These types of endurance activities tend to be
fuelled by the body's fat stores and are therefore great for people who
want to lose fat. They also help improve the functioning of your heart
and lungs, and help make muscles fit and more efficient.

Anaerobic exercises do not have such heavy and immediate oxygen
needs. These exercises focus on muscle strength and require surges of
power, rather than endurance. The most common anerobic exercise is
called resistance or strength training, in which your muscles push or
pull against a resisting force, such as dumbbells, free weights or
resistive bands. The result is that lean body mass gets built up so that
metabolism burns at its optimal level. These types of power-surge
activities are mainly fueled by glucose, not fat stores.

Ideally, every woman – regardless of body shape – should do both
aerobic exercise and strength training to lose fat and get maximal
health benefits. Women lose more subcutaneous and visceral fat when
they do both types of exercise than when they do just one type. Plus,
the general health effects are improved with both exercise types – when
women walk and do strength training, their insulin sensitivity increases
even more than if they only walk. It is the combination of both kinds

of exercise that allows apple-shaped women to lose girth from their waists and decrease their disease risk factors.

Pear-shaped women will want to do aerobic exercise to lose fat and to do strength training to help build metabolism. As I discussed in chapter 12, pear-shaped women have a generally lower metabolism than apple-shaped women. Part of the reason is that apple-shaped women have more androgen, giving them greater muscle mass and higher metabolism. If you want to raise your metabolism, you'll have to build muscle mass through strength training. (Please note that greater muscle mass doesn't mean having a build like Arnold Schwarzenegger or The Rock – it just means more lean tissue than fat tissue in a feminine package.)

Pear-shaped women should also note that exercises that put pressure on bones – what are called *weight-bearing exercises* – help prevent and even reverse bone density loss of osteoporosis, regardless of the woman's age or the status of her bones before she starts exercising. One example of a weight-bearing exercise is walking, because one foot is always on the ground – at every moment at least one foot is bearing the weight of your whole body. This is why walking, is such an all-around fabulous exercise – it is both aerobic and weight bearing, and it requires a minimum of preparation and equipment. Swimming, on the other hand, is a terrific aerobic exercise, but it is not a weight-bearing exercise because you are held up by the water.

Weight-bearing exercises help prevent and even reverse bone density loss of osteoporosis, regardless of the woman's age or the status of her bones before she starts exercising.

All resistance or strength training is weight-bearing, because the activity is defined by the pushing or pulling of weight or a force. So resistance exercises help build bones. A programme of just two days per week of six low-intensity exercises per session is enough to increase bone mineral density in postmenopausal women. Of course, the more weight-bearing exercise you do, the stronger your bones will be, but even a minimal effort will help prevent bone loss. This is not a major time commitment, just a nice addition to your repertoire.

REASONS VERSUS EXCUSES

So, now that you know why exercise is important and what it can do for you, do you want to exercise? Or, let me put it a different way: are you willing to exercise to improve your health and lose girth from your apple- or pear-zone?

If your answer is no, then there is really nothing anyone can do to persuade you to put on your trainers and sweatpants and get moving. Every day we make decisions that have health consequences. If your decision is not to exercise, then you also forfeit your right to complain about gaining weight. If you don't exercise, you will gain weight over the years, I guarantee it. If this is your choice, then embrace it. Own it. Stop making excuses for why you aren't exercising and just say that you have made a conscious decision not to exercise.

On the other hand, if your answer is yes, and you checked off one or more of the reason boxes at the beginning of this chapter, let's try to fix some of those problems.

No Time

This is the toughest hurdle. Time is at a premium for everyone, and the thought of squeezing in one more activity is enough to send some women right over the edge. I won't tell you to wake up earlier because most of the women I know don't get enough sleep as it is. There are three things you can try.

First, decide which other activity can be ignored for a while. For example, if you spend 30 minutes or more vacuuming your house every day, try vacuuming every other day instead, and exercise on the days you don't vacuum. If you have a favourite television show you have to watch, videotape it and watch it while you are doing your resistance exercises. Carve out whatever time you can to take care of your body's needs.

Second, make the routine as easy as possible. You don't need to put on special workout clothes or set up equipment every time you want to exercise. Walking can be done anytime while wearing just about any type of clothing. All you need is a pair of comfortable trainers or walking shoes, and you can go. Don't waste time getting ready, just move.

Third, look for ways to make common activities more active. This goes against the grain for many of us because we've learned to conserve energy. Take two trips up the stairs with the laundry instead of one, do leg stretches while brushing your teeth, or walk around the house while talking on the phone instead of plopping on the couch. If you don't already own a mobile phone, buy one and consider it an investment as you walk and talk your way to better health. All these little activities add up to burned calories. But in the end, it comes down to priorities. If you lose your health, nothing else will get done, either. Everyone is busy, but the women who know how important it is to take care of themselves make time for exercise.

Hate Exercising

If you hate exercising then you simply haven't found the right activity. Most kids naturally love to run around. They jump rope, play tag or hopscotch, and can spend hours outdoors. We have to regain that love of movement. It's in us – we just have to rediscover what it is we like to do. I would love to see adult women take up jumping rope again and to have the same kinds of contests and trick exhibitions that kids have. If jumping isn't your thing, what about slow, calm yoga; or gentle tai chi; or cool, languid swimming; or skating, cycling or hiking? One 43-year-old woman I know hated exercise until she started attending her children's tae kwon do classes. She was hooked as soon as she got her yellow belt and felt that pride of strength and accomplishment no other physical activity had been able to give her.

It Hurts

It used to be that the motto of exercise fanatics was 'No Pain, No Gain'. Well, scientists have discovered that that's not strictly true. However, 'No Exercise, No Pain', is true and that's exactly what many people did – avoided the pain by avoiding the exercise.

Exercise shouldn't hurt. If it hurts, you are doing something wrong.

Exercise shouldn't hurt. If it hurts, you are doing something wrong. You can become stronger and healthier without feeling bad physically. Think about the last time you took a pleasant walk. Maybe it was on a long stretch of beach, or through the streets of a city you were visiting, or even walking around a zoo or a park with your family. That was exercise. If it was a much longer walk than you were used to, you may have felt a little muscle stiffness the next day or two, but that fades as you do more walking.

The problem is that many women talk themselves out of exercising because they fear the pain. One researcher asked women to predict how much physical discomfort they would feel during exercise. Then they exercised, and afterward the researcher asked them how much discomfort they actually felt. For the most part, the women overpredicted how awful exercise would be – it turned out to be not nearly as bad as they had imagined. We don't know why this happens, but it tells us that we need to stop dreading the activity. We need to remind ourselves that it won't be horrible, and in fact, it might actually be fun. I know that even if I'm having a low-energy day and the exercise itself isn't fun, I always feel really good afterward – healthy, happy, powerful and confident. On days when it is tough to get going, the anticipation of this exercise afterglow is my motivation.

Forgetfulness or Different Priorities

This usually goes along with not having enough time. If exercise isn't near the top of your priority list, it will never get done. Taking care of your health has to come before taking care of the laundry or the dishes. It's up to you to decide how important losing fat and preventing heart disease is to you. If it's not important, then stop making excuses and just admit that you choose not to exercise. Forgetfulness, on the other hand, is a little easier to deal with. If you are not used to exercising every day, then it is more likely to slip your mind when you get busy, despite your best intentions. The solution here is to put your trainers in the middle of the kitchen table, or blocking the doorway, or anywhere else you won't be able to miss.

No Equipment

Having a treadmill or elliptical machine is great for people who use them, but most women end up turning the equipment into very expensive clotheslines. You don't need equipment. You need motivation, trainers, and – at most – a set of Thera-Band exercise bands for resistance training (see page 305).

It's Just a Fad

Actually, it isn't a bad thing to have so many exercise options. Different people respond to different activities. Some women get bored walking alone, while others can't stand going indoors to take classes in a gym. Some women like the variety of having a new 'fad' every few years, but others like the stability of doing the same activity for the rest of their lives. You don't have to latch on to every new training method that comes out, but feel free to try them all to see if any are right for you. Most instructors or gyms will allow you to take a free or reduced-cost class before signing up for a long-term commitment. Look around, sample the variety and have fun.

Low Return on Your Time Investment

Exercise is never without benefit, even if you cannot see it. You may never lose a kilo, but your body is still getting healthier, performing at a more optimal level. Remember that 36 per cent lower risk of death in women who exercise even minimally? Are you looking for a bigger return than that?

Not Safe

This is a major issue for many women, and there is no way for me to minimise the threat. If you feel unsafe, you will never enjoy exercising. If possible, move your exercise indoors by buying a treadmill or joining a gym – there are many low-cost options, so look around. Walk briskly around the inside of a shopping mall – you won't be alone, and the environment is usually safe. If you work outside the home, find out if your workplace offers any incentive for gym membership or if there are fitness classes offered on the premises. Band together with others from your neighbourhood and walk as a group. If you walk at night, always wear light-coloured clothing and carry a torch so that drivers in passing cars can see you – and you can see what or who is coming toward you. Never put your safety at risk.

No One Ever Told You Why Exercise Is Important

Now you know.

Confusion or Frustration

The rest of this chapter tells you exactly what to do and how to do it.

THE APPLES AND PEARS EXERCISE PROGRAMME

Important note: if you have not been exercising regularly and are about to start a new activity programme, have a physical examination just to be certain that it is medically safe for you to exercise. Your doctor will be thrilled at your initiative, and will probably be more than willing to answer all your exercise-related questions and concerns. Apple-shaped women with risk factors for heart disease should probably have a stress test. Your doctor will be able to make the appropriate recommendations.

If you are not used to exercising, start with the schedule for beginners. This will give you an easier transition into a more active lifestyle, with less of a risk of injury. Perform the exercises at your own pace, and with an intensity or resistance level that is most comfortable for you. Whatever you do, *don't push it.* I would rather you underdo it than overdo it. If you overdo exercise, you run the risk of pulling a muscle, straining a ligament, or even becoming so sore that exercise will be impossible for days or even weeks afterward. If you underdo it, you can always make up for it next time. Exercise is supposed to make you strong, not crippled with pain. If you do become injured, rest up for a few days, then try again with a lower intensity.

EXERCISE SCHEDULE – BEGINNERS

Monday: 30 to 45 minutes of an aerobic exercise

Tuesday: 6 different resistance band exercises, two sets of 8 repetitions each

Wednesday: 30 to 45 minutes of an aerobic exercise

Thursday: 6 different resistance band exercises, two sets of 8 repetitions each

Friday: 30 to 45 minutes of an aerobic exercise

Weekend: A fun activity of your choice – golfing, tennis, hiking, skating, skiing, swimming, playing with your children or grandchildren or even walking around a mall

If you are currently active, or if you have been following the beginners' schedule for at least four weeks and want to step up to the next level, use the schedule for optimal exercise.

EXERCISE SCHEDULE – OPTIMAL

Monday: 45 to 60 minutes of an aerobic exercise

Tuesday: 6 different resistance band exercises, three sets of 12 repetitions each

Wednesday: 45 to 60 minutes of an aerobic exercise

Thursday: 6 different resistance band exercises, three sets of 12 repetitions each

Friday: 45 to 60 minutes of an aerobic exercise

Weekend: A fun activity of your choice

These are the current guidelines for optimal weight loss. Studies show that if you exercise for 30 minutes a day, 5 days per week, that is usually enough to keep you from getting fatter. Remember, we all tend to put on weight as we get older, and this penchant for padding escalates after menopause. If you are exercising moderately and not seeing any weight loss, it may be that you are simply stopping the extra kilos from creeping up. That's important, too. But if you want to lose girth, you'll have to step up the overall amount of exercise you do. For that you'll need *45 to 60 minutes of moderate exercise three to seven days per week.*

Exercise works in a dose-dependent way – the more exercise you do, the more impressive the results will be. If you do a little exercise, you'll lose a little fat. If you do a lot of exercise, you'll lose a lot of fat. If you walk seven days a week, you'll slim faster than if you walk three days per week. It is totally within your power to choose the amount of fat you keep on your body simply by choosing the amount of exercise you do. I'm not talking about a quick fix – weight that is lost quickly always seems to find its way back. But if you exercise regularly – even just 45 minutes of walking per day – you *will* lose fat.

One important note about exercise and weight loss: most people experience a slight decrease in appetite after exercise. This is nothing to be concerned about – it is perfectly normal and desirable if you want to lose girth. However, some people find themselves eating more after exercise, often because they feel a need to reward themselves for being 'good', or because they think that exercise entitles them to eat more. Don't fall into this trap. The point of exercise is to burn the extra calories that have already found a home in your fat cells. If you eat more, then your efforts will go to 'waist'.

AEROBIC EXERCISE

My favourite aerobic exercise is walking. You can do it anywhere, for as long or as short as you like. All you need is a sturdy, supportive pair of shoes and a safe path. If you walk on a street, walk on the right side, facing traffic – this allows you to see oncoming cars and take action in case of an emergency.

Start by walking at a pace that is comfortable for you – not so slow that you don't feel challenged, but not so fast that you can't catch your breath. A good rule of thumb is that you should be able to hold a conversation without panting. If you are just beginning to get active, work your way up to the recommended 45 minutes. Walk until you feel tired but not exhausted. Add five minutes each week until you are able to walk 45 minutes comfortably. The longer you stick with the programme, the easier it will become. As your walking pace becomes too comfortable, pick up the pace a little to get a better cardio-respiratory workout.

For fun – if you are interested – buy a pedometer to monitor how many steps you walk in a day. Experts say that we need 10,000 steps from dawn to bedtime to maintain fitness. I don't like to be so rigid about numbers. When I put on my pedometer I'm always surprised by how much, or how little, I move during a particular day. It's easy to over- or underestimate exactly how many steps I take. You can purchase a pedometer any place where sporting goods are sold. Unless you like cool gadgets with a lot of unnecessary options, opt for the least expensive model, which will cost about £5.00.

If possible, take a headset and a Walkman or iPod so you can listen to music. Research has shown that people who listen to music exercise longer and feel less discomfort while walking.

Running and jogging are good aerobic exercises, but they are not as good for bones as walking because there are times when both feet are off the ground so they are not consistently weight-bearing. Plus, running isn't an option for many women because our hip and leg structure creates a greater risk of knee injury or pain. Other good aerobic activities are hiking, swimming, basketball, skating, tennis, dancing, aerobic classes, cycling, spinning, elliptical stepping or anything else that keeps you moving consistently for a long time.

RESISTANCE TRAINING

For strength or resistance training, I recommend using Thera-Band resistance bands. This is a system of large elasticated bands that allow you to perform hundreds of exercises for all muscle groups with the same piece of equipment. These are the same colourful bands used by athletes and by people who need physical therapy during rehabilitation to increase muscle strength. The band colour relates to the resistance level of the elastic; with each step up, the same exercise becomes more challenging. From lightest to heaviest the levels are yellow, red, green, blue, black, silver.

I like the elastic bands instead of hand weights (dumbbells) or free weights because they are less likely to cause injury. Plus, they are portable and easy to store. They are so light and compact that each band can easily fit in the zip compartment of a handbag or briefcase. Best of all, they are affordable. You can purchase a three-pack of six-foot Light Bands (yellow, red, green) or a three-pack of six-foot Heavy Bands (blue, black, silver) for about £10.50. Nonlatex bands are available, but they are more expensive.

To order one of these sets, contact PHYSIO-MED Services (01457 860444; www.physio-med.com). Ask for the Thera-Band Light Band Kit and/or Heavy Band Kit. (Please note: Thera-Band resistance bands have been well tested and are quality controlled. This is the brand used by professionals around the world. Other companies produce imitation bands, but I cannot recommend them.)

I've included my top 12 favourite elastic resistance exercises and some bonus exercises, which together allow for total body conditioning. Do six on the first day of your workout, and a different six on the second day. You can add a third day of resistance training if you enjoy it. For this third day, choose any six exercises you like. (For additional exercises, see the recommendations at www.thera-bandacademy.com.)

Here's how to get the most from resistance training:

◆ Follow the pictures and written instructions carefully, noting the precise location of the band in relation to the model's body.

◆ Perform each exercise with slow, controlled movements.

◆ Keep your back and neck stable as you perform the exercise. Posture is very important. If you strain, or twist or arch your back, you could cause injury. If you cannot complete the full range of motion without changing your posture, go to a lower-resistance band.

◆ Keep the band tension relatively tight – it should not go entirely slack, even when you are in the starting position.

◆ Make sure both sides of your body get equal time.

◆ Try to coordinate your breathing to the motion of the exercise. Breathe out (exhale) while doing the straining part of the exercise; breathe in as you relax.

◆ After each set of 8 or 12 repetitions, rest for one minute, then do the next set. Finish all sets of a single exercise before moving on to the next exercise.

◆ You should be able to do the sets without pain, while still feeling that your muscles have been challenged. If the exercise is too easy, then move to the next heavier resistance band colour. If the exercise is too hard to complete, or if it causes pain, move to a lighter resistance band colour. If you feel persistent pain while doing an exercise, see your doctor.

◆ You can change band colours between sets for a better workout. When you are moving from one level of difficulty to the next, you can start with a heavier resistance band for the first set or two, then move to a lighter resistance band for the next set as you get tired.

◆ Your goal is to be able to move up the resistance levels to the heaviest grade. Do this at your own pace – it is not a race. Enjoy the sense of accomplishment that comes from moving up from one level to the next.

Important note: Always secure the end of the band so it will not come loose. If the exercise calls for you to step on one end, keep your foot firmly on the band. If the exercise calls for you to secure the band to a door, the best and safest way to do this is to purchase a specific door anchor. Thera-Band also make a door anchor and handles, available from PHYSIO-MED Services (see opposite) at about £7.00 each, including VAT but not p&p. Alternatively, you can make a secure knot in the band at the end that needs to be anchored, then close the knot in a door so that the round ball of the knot acts as an anchor. (Always inspect the bands for tears or wear, which may cause them to break unexpectedly.)

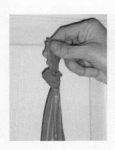 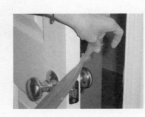 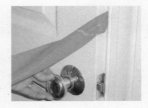

RESISTANCE EXERCISES

E X E R C I S E 1
Super Abdominal Crunch
(Stomach)

Anchor the band in a door, about doorknob height. Lie on your back with your head closest to the door. Grip the band, holding your arms straight up, perpendicular to the floor (see figure 12a). Pull the band forward and down, towards the space between your knees, while raising your shoulder blades off the ground. Keep your elbows and neck straight (see figure 12b). Hold for a count of two, then slowly return to the starting position. Repeat for 8 or 12 repetitions.

Bonus exercise (not pictured): To exercise your oblique abdominal muscles, pull the band to the sides instead of straight down. From the same starting position, pull the band towards your left knee while lifting your right shoulder slightly. Hold for a count of two, then slowly return. Do 12 repetitions. Then repeat on the other side – pulling the band towards your right knee while lifting your left shoulder slightly.

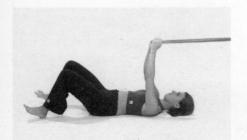

Fig. 12a. Super Crunch, Start

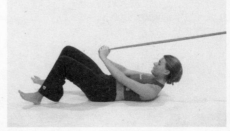

Fig. 12b. Super Crunch, End

EXERCISE 2
Cross Pull
(Chest, Shoulders)

Anchor the band in a door, about doorknob height. Stand with your left side towards the door. Grasp the end of the band with your left hand, palm facing forward (see figure 13a). Pull the band low across your body, towards your right thigh. Keep your elbow straight. Your palm will end up facing your thigh (see figure 13b). Hold for a count of two, then return to the starting position. Repeat for 8 or 12 repetitions. Turn and repeat on the other side.

Bonus exercise (not pictured): From the same starting position, pull the band high across your body until your hand is even with your right shoulder. Keep your elbow straight. Do 8 or 12 repetitions, then repeat on the other side.

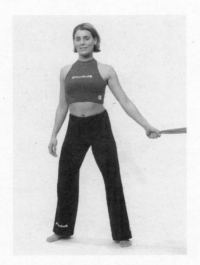

Fig. 13a. Cross Pull, Start

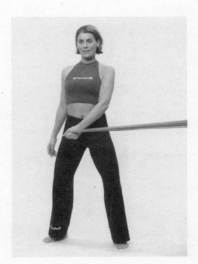

Fig. 13b. Cross Pull, End

EXERCISE 3
X-Raise
(Shoulders, Arms)

Stand with your feet shoulder-width apart on the middle of a 1.8m (6ft) band. Bend your knees slightly. Cross the band in front of your body and wrap both ends around your hands. Face your palms forward (see figure 14a). Lift your arms away from your side to an overhead position, keeping your elbows straight and your palms up (see figure 14b). Hold for a count of two, then slowly return. Repeat for 12 repetitions. Note – in this exercise, it is critical to keep your back straight. If you find yourself arching your back, move to a lower resistance band.

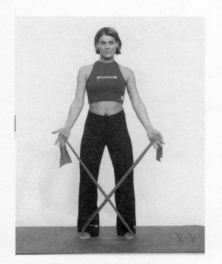

Fig. 14a. X-raise, Start

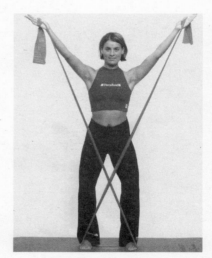

Fig. 14b. X-raise, End

EXERCISE 4
Strong Arms
(Biceps)

Step forward with one foot and loop the middle of the band under that foot. Grip an end of the band in each hand. Start with your arms extended straight downward towards your forward foot (see figure 15a). The band should already have some tension – if it is too loose, wrap some length around your hands until there is a light tension. Pull both ends of the band towards your chest by bending your elbows. Do not move your shoulders or your body. When your hands are even with your chest (see figure 15b), hold for a count of two, then return to the starting position. Do 12 repetitions.

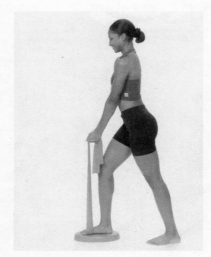

Fig. 15a. Strong Arms, Start

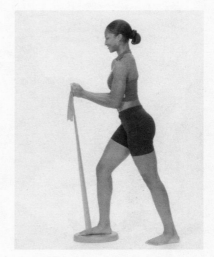

Fig. 15b. Strong Arms, End

EXERCISE 5

Flying

(Chest, Back, Arms)

Anchor the middle of a band at the top of a door. (Tie a knot in the middle of the band and anchor in the same manner as illustrated on page 307.) Face the door and step forward with one foot. You should be at least 60cm (2ft) away from the door. Grip an end of the band in each hand. Start with your arms straight at shoulder level, palms facing inward (see figure 16a). Keep your elbows straight throughout the exercise. Pull both ends of the band down, between your thighs (see figure 16b). When you reach your forward thigh, stop, hold for a count of two, then return to the starting position. Repeat for 12 repetitions.

Bonus exercise (not pictured): From the same starting position (see figure 16a), keeping elbows straight, pull both ends of the band out to your sides (see figure 16c). Hold for a count of two, then return to the starting position. Repeat for 12 repetitions.

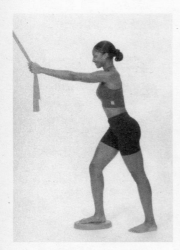

Fig. 16a. Flying, Start

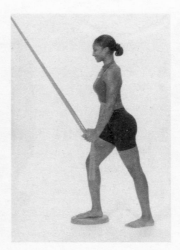

Fig. 16b. Flying, Middle

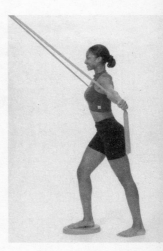

Fig. 16c. Flying, End

312 SOLUTIONS

EXERCISE 6
Push Out
(Chest, Arms)

Loop the middle of the band around your back and under your arms. Grip an end of the band in each hand. Start with elbows bent and close to your body, hands at the level of your chest, palms facing inward (see figure 17a). Extend your hands forward by straightening your elbows (see figure 17b). When your arms are fully extended, hold for a count of two, then return to the starting position. Repeat for 12 repetitions.

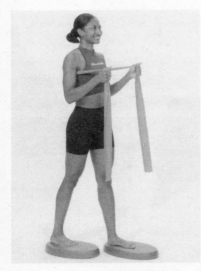

Fig. 17a. Push Out, Start

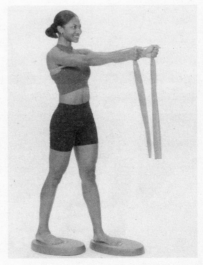

Fig. 17b. Push Out, End

EXERCISE 7
Cross Kick
(Inner Thighs)

Loop the band and anchor both ends in a door about 15cm (6in) from the floor. Standing with your left side closest to the door, put your left leg in the loop of the band. Move just far enough away from the door so that when you put your weight on your right leg, your left leg is pulled slightly outward towards the door. Place your weight on your right leg. Keep your stomach and buttocks muscles tight and your back straight (see figure 18a). Slowly move your left leg away from the door towards your body, keeping your knees straight. As your left leg crosses in front of your right leg (see figure 18b), hold for a count of two, then slowly return. Repeat for 12 repetitions. Then repeat with the right leg.

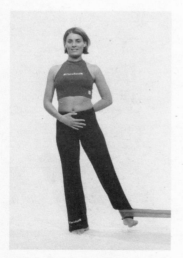
Fig. 18a. Cross Kick, Start

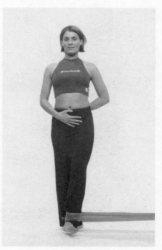
Fig. 18b. Cross Kick, End

EXERCISE 8
Kick Out
(Outer Thighs)

Loop the band and anchor both ends in a door about 15cm (6in) from the floor. Standing with your left side closest to the door, put your right leg in the loop of the band. Move just far enough away from the door so that when you put your feet together, there is a slight tension on the band. (Your left leg should be in front of the band.) Place your weight on your left leg. Keep your stomach and buttocks muscles tight and your back straight (see figure 19a). Slowly move your right leg outward, away from the door, keeping your knees straight (see figure 19b). Hold the position farthest from your body for a count of two, then slowly return. Repeat for 12 repetitions. Then repeat with the left leg.

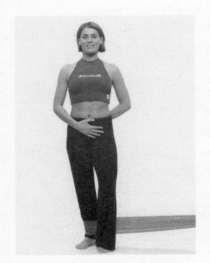

Fig. 19a. Kick Out, Start

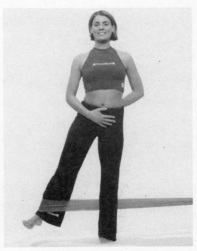

Fig. 19b. Kick Out, End

Thigh Strengthener

(Thighs, Balance)

If you have a difficulty standing on one foot, hold on to a wall or chair while performing this exercise.

Anchor both ends of a band in a door, about 15cm (6in) from the floor. Face the door. Put your right ankle in the loop and move backward away from the door until your right leg is extended forward, pulled by the band (see figure 20a). Bend your knee to pull your right foot towards your body (see figure 20b). Hold for a count of two, then return to the starting position. Repeat for 12 repetitions. Repeat using your left leg.

Bonus exercise (not pictured): From the same starting position (see figure 20a), pull your right leg towards your body *without bending your knee*. Pull until you cannot pull any farther (this may be even with or behind your left leg). Hold for a count of two, then return to starting position. Repeat for 12 repetitions. Repeat using your left leg.

Bonus exercise (not pictured): Anchor the band in the same manner. Face away from the door. Put your left ankle in the loop. Move far enough away from the door so that when your feet are together, you feel a tension on the band around your ankle. Put your weight on your right leg. Keeping your knee straight, extend your left leg forward so that your foot is pointed away from the door and away from your body. Hold for a count of two, then return to starting position. Repeat for 12 repetitions. Repeat using your right leg.

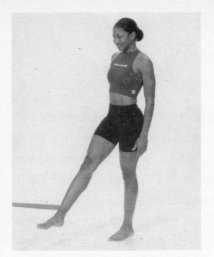
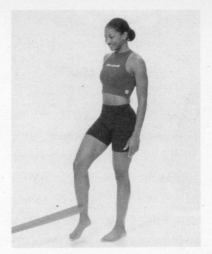

Fig. 20a. Thigh Strengthener, Start   Fig. 20b. Thigh Strengthener, End

Leg Curls

(Hamstrings)

Anchor both ends of a band in a door, about 15cm (6in) from the floor. Lie down on your stomach, with your head facing away from the door. Loop the band around your right ankle. Move far enough away so that there is moderate tension on the band (see figure 21a). Pull the band by bending your knee. Be certain to keep your back stable. Stop when your shin is perpendicular to the floor (see figure 21b), hold for a count of two. Return to the starting position. Repeat for 12 repetitions. Repeat with your left leg.

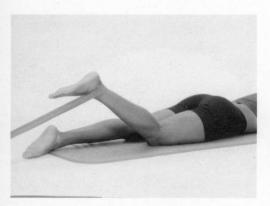

Fig. 21a. Leg Curls, Start

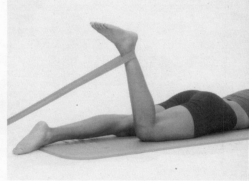

Fig. 21b. Leg Curls, End

EXERCISE 11
Back Kick
(Back, Buttocks)

Get on your hands and knees. Loop the middle of the 1.8m (6ft) band around your right foot and grip an end with each hand (put your hands back on the floor). Keep your eyes focused on the floor, and keep your neck and back straight (see figure 22a). Slowly extend your right leg until your back and your leg are in a straight line (see figure 22b). Hold for a count of two, then slowly return to the starting position. Repeat for 12 repetitions. Repeat with the left leg.

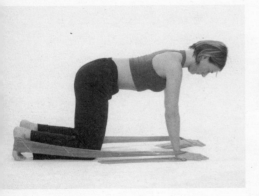

Fig. 22a. Back Kick, Start

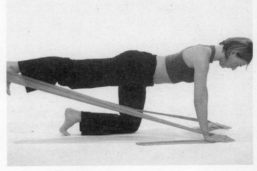

Fig. 22b. Back Kick, End

EXERCISE 12
Reverse Crunch
(Back, Abdominals, Arms)

Sit on the floor with your legs together, straight out in front of you. Loop the band around both feet, cross the band in front of your body, and grip an end in each hand. Hold your hands against your stomach (see figure 23a). Lean backward slightly, keeping your back and neck straight. Your arms and hands should remain in position (see figure 23b). (The pull should come from your body, not your arms.) Hold the end position for a count of two, then slowly return to the starting position. Repeat for 12 repetitions.

Bonus exercise (not pictured): From the same starting position, extend your arms towards your toes. Tighten up the tension on the band. Keep your back straight and pull your elbows back so that your hands end up at your waist. (The pull is coming from your arms, not your body.) Hold the end position for a count of two, then slowly return to the starting position. Repeat for 12 repetitions.

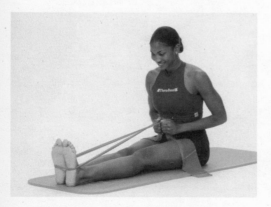 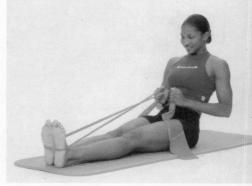

Fig. 23a. Reverse Crunch, Start   Fig. 23b. Reverse Crunch, End

CHAPTER 14

The Power of Body Shape

I hope I have given you a new way to think about yourself, your body and your health. My major goal in writing this book was to provide all women with the information and tools they need to stay as healthy as possible, now and for the rest of their lives.

This book grew out of my love for my sister Millie, and my urgent wish that I could travel back in time and undo the damage that undiagnosed type 2 diabetes had done to her body. So much could have been done differently, by her, by her doctors. She didn't need to suffer painful neuropathy. She didn't need to wait years before taking control of the risk factors that eventually added up to diabetes and its complications. But back then, the signs pointing to body shape as a risk measurement tool weren't that strong. We didn't have the language or the vocabulary to talk about visceral fat and waist-to-hip ratio. And we certainly didn't have enough of the medical research puzzle pieced together to see clearly what picture was taking shape. I can let that go, forgive myself and her doctors, because the basic knowledge just wasn't there yet. Today is different.

Today, I make sure that the women I treat and meet in my travels understand the powerful influence body shape has on nearly every aspect of women's health – from self-esteem to stress reactions; from reproductive capability to symptoms and treatment of menopause; from stiffening arteries to crumbling bones. The apple-shaped women who are my patients get clear instructions very early on about how to prevent heart disease, the metabolic syndrome, and all the other disorders that arise from excess visceral fat. My pear-shaped patients are asked about body image and sent for bone density tests in their mid-40s; they receive advice about healthy balanced diets and exercise and are warned of the risks and foolishness of radical and quick weight loss. But that's just me. There is a whole world of physicians out there who are not yet tuned in to the body shape-wellness connection. This means that, as of this moment, you may have more information about the power of body shape than your doctor does. It is both your blessing and your challenge.

JOINING HANDS

As this book is being written, scientists are hard at work trying to decode the human genome so that they can understand what our DNA tells us about our individual disease risks. Someday, probably not in our lifetimes, people will be able to have a few of their body cells analysed and their entire physiologic inheritance will be revealed. Then, they will be able to receive targeted therapies custom designed for their specific needs. That kind of amazing technology probably won't tell us a whole lot more than body shape can. And really, body shape is even a better medical tool because it is a health measure everyone can afford. Every woman can learn from a tape measure, regardless of her insurance, income or education level.

As wonderful as technology can be, ultra-fast computed tomography, magnetic resonance imaging, genetic testing and even some blood tests are available only to those who can pay, or who have the medical sophistication or knowledge to ask for them. But we all love our new gadgets, and the medical community is no different. But just because a piece of equipment is new and expensive doesn't mean it is the best tool for the job. With a simple tape measure, there are no health risks and no concern about excessive or unnecessary testing. But in order to be valuable, the tape measure has to be used. Few doctors take the initiative to measure waist and hip circumference, which means that body shape is still not part of the general medical dialogue. It should be, and I predict it will be very soon.

You can be a part of that transition. I have devoted much of my career to teaching doctors and patients how to collaborate effectively to create the best possible environment for pursuing health. Not that long ago, the doctor was always in control of medical decision making. Now, we all need to be more intimately involved in the process of health care. And the best way to do that is to join hands with your doctor and work together, to form a partnership with the primary purpose of making you the healthiest you can be.

I know the idea of partnering with a doctor is foreign and even frightening to many people. Women tell me how they cower before their physicians, often afraid to speak up, afraid to trust their instincts, afraid they will be wrong. Too many women leave their confidence behind in the waiting room (along with the two-year-old copy of *Ideal Home*). But when we insist on being collaborative partners, the results can be just this side of miraculous. For example, I recently met Wendy, who told me about her trouble getting a physician to take her health concerns seriously. After hearing about the power of body shape, Wendy did some research and figured out that she must have polycystic ovary syndrome (PCOS). She had finally put all the puzzle pieces of her health together – her apple shape, excess facial hair, irregular periods and inability to lose weight. She was very excited when she presented her findings to her doctor. He did the blood work and discovered that although the numbers were a little off, they were still in the normal range, and therefore he would not give her a diagnosis of PCOS. Nor would he prescribe or even suggest treatment for her symptoms. The results of her blood tests didn't fit his rigid schema of disease, so Wendy and her concerns were dismissed. It was a cookery book approach to doctoring that didn't end up helping the patient.

Wendy switched doctors, summoned the courage to explain her concerns again, and this time it worked. The doctor really listened to her, worked with her to understand her symptoms and what might be causing them. This new doctor considered that Wendy could be right. Diseases come in all shapes and sizes, and they rarely fit the textbook perfectly. This wise doctor also knew that women often know when something is wrong in their bodies, and most of them don't complain for no reason. Wendy's doctor agreed to treat her for PCOS, trusting in the doctor-patient partnership, willing to give Wendy a voice in her own health care. She was put on a medication to help her lose weight and improve her insulin resistance. Almost immediately, Wendy started losing fat from around her waist, and she even started having more regular periods. Both she and her new doctor know to keep their eyes open for signs of other disorders that might pop up in the future because of her extreme apple shape, and they are both ready to take whatever steps are needed to keep her healthy. For the first time in her life, Wendy feels as though her health is under control.

INDIVIDUALIZED HEALTH GOALS

Now that you know how important body shape is for your future health, the next step is to get your doctor involved at that same level. Talk with your doctor about any concerns you might have about body weight. Bring a tape measure to your next appointment, and make sure your measurements get noted in your file. Immediately following this chapter, beginning on page 328, you will find the Body Shape Health Logs for apple- and pear-shaped women. These forms outline the tests I specifically recommend for women, based on body shape. Bring the form to your doctor so that she understands exactly what you are looking for, and then work together to determine your personal target goals for each item.

Of course, we all have an ultimate goal of having 'normal' numbers, but if your numbers are currently off the charts, your intermediate goals may be different. For example, if you are an apple-shaped woman, then I would like your target goal for waist circumference to be just 5cm (2in) smaller than what it is today. Although many scientists recommend an ideal waist circumference of less than 80cm (32in), that number may be too large for some very small apple-shaped women, leaving them with significant amounts of excess visceral fat. For other women, 80cm (32in) will be an unrealistic goal, and I don't think it is fair to burden anyone with such an overwhelming task. A loss of 5cm (2in) is a wonderful target goal. Work with your doctor to set targets for all the other tests on the forms.

YOUR HEALTHY FUTURE

It all comes down to you.

Body shape is a potent predictor of future health, the basic road map of our life's journey, but it doesn't tell us everything. Diet, exercise, stress, sleep and other choices make up the detours, side trips, and pit stops. Where you end up depends on all these factors together.

My goal has been to help you move away from the one-size-fits-all diet plans and wellness gimmicks – to understand that it all comes down to your choices, your dreams of your future and your life priorities. I hope that this book has given you the tools you need to make these life decisions from a position of strength and wisdom.

My personal wish for the pear-shaped women of the world is that you learn to appreciate that your body is perfect – Nature's perfection. It is doing what it should be doing by storing fat in case of need and protecting you from early disease. Your pear-zone fat will help keep you healthy for years to come. Try not to waste these years by being at war with your body. Stop looking for a 'magic bullet' or miracle treatment to get rid of your shape. Ultimately, I wish you the peace of mind that comes from personal confidence.

My personal wish for the apple-shaped women of the world is that you understand your disease risks without becoming anxious or depressed. Instead, be glad that this information is available and that you have discovered this crystal ball while there is still time to make a difference. Remember that one of the main messages of the research is that it is never too late to make a difference. Look at the information about body shape as the 'Aha!' moment that gets you finally to join a gym, eat healthily and just generally take care of yourself. If your family's legacy is one of heart disease or diabetes, I hope that this information makes you feel hopeful, confident and inspired to action. Apple-shaped women have tremendous strength and fortitude, and my ultimate wish is that you have a long, healthy life in which to enjoy these blessings.

YOUR BODY SHAPE HEALTH LOG

Using your Body Shape Health Log will help you (and your doctor) determine how well you are doing in meeting your personal target goals for particular risk factors. It can also help you spot important trends in test results that may signal an impending change in your health.

I have included separate logs for apple- and pear-shaped women so that you can track the tests that are most important for you. Because your medical and family history is unique, you and your doctor will need to work together to select your specific target goals for each test. Here are the simple steps for using the Body Shape Health Log.

I. Select the Body Shape Health Log for your shape. Women with a waist-hip ratio greater than 0.80 should use the form for apple-shaped women on page 328. Women with a waist-hip ratio of 0.80 or lower should use the form for pear-shaped women on page 329. (If you are a pear-shaped woman but have been diagnosed with a metabolic disorder, type 2 diabetes, or heart disease, you should also use the form for apple-shaped women because you'll need to track a different set of tests.) You can use the form in the book or make a photocopy. The form is also available online at www. applesandpears.org.

2. Remember, women who take only 5cm (2in) off their waists will dramatically improve their disease risk factors. If your waist circumference is larger than 76cm (30in), make your first target goal for waist circumference 5cm (2in) smaller than your current waist size. Measure your waist circumference and recalculate your waist-hip ratio every 6 months.

3. Take your Body Shape Health Log to your next doctor appointment. Discuss with your doctor which of the tests and procedures yo may need, and how often they should be repeated. Write down the target goals agreed upon by you and your doctor in the far right-hand column. Ask your doctor to send a copy of all test results to your home. Once the tests are performed, write your results in the first column. Follow-up test results can be tracked by recording them in the next column. (Be sure to put the date of the test at the top of the appropriate column.)

4. Bring your Body Shape Health Log to every doctor visit to make sure it is up to date and to revise target goals if necessary.

Body Shape Health Log (for apple-shaped women)

Name _____ Date of Birth _____

DATE:						Target Goal
Waist/Hip Ratio						
Waist Circumference						
Height/Weight						
BMI (body mass index)						
Blood Pressure						
Blood Glucose						
Haemoglobin A1C						
Urine for Protein						
Total Cholesterol						
HDL (good)						
LDL (bad)						
Triglycerides						
C-Reactive Protein (CRP)						
TSH (thyroid function)						
EKG						
Cardiac Stress Test						
Vision/Dilated Eye Exam						
Breast Exam						
Mammogram						
Rectal Exam						
Colon Cancer Check						
Pelvic Exam						
Smear Test						
HPV and Smear Test						

Other exams/tests to discuss with your doctor include: Total Skin Exam, Dental Exam, Bone Density Exam, Complete Blood Count and Basic Metabolic Profile.

an apple-shaped woman = waist/hip ratio > 0.80

Body Shape Health Log (for pear-shaped women)

Name _____ Date of Birth _____

DATE:					Target Goal
Waist/Hip Ratio					
Waist Circumference					
Height/Weight					
BMI (body mass index)					
Blood Pressure					
Blood Glucose					
Total Cholesterol					
HDL (good)					
LDL (bad)					
Triglycerides					
TSH (thyroid function)					
EKG					
Eye Exam					
Breast Exam					
Mammogram					
Rectal Exam					
Colon Cancer Check					
Pelvic Exam					
Smear Test					
HPV and Smear Test					
Bone Density Exam					

Other exams/tests to discuss with your doctor include: Total Skin Exam, Dental Exam, Complete Blood Count and Basic Metabolic Profile.

a pear-shaped woman = waist/hip ratio ≤ 0.80

© 2004 Marie Savard, M.D.
www.applesandpears.org

Selected References

Chapter 1

Bonora, E., S. Del Prato, R. C. Bonadonna, et al. Total body fat content and fat topography are associated differently with in vivo glucose metabolism in nonobese and obese nondiabetic women. *Diabetes* 1992;41(9):1151–59.

Després, J. P., A. Nadeau, A. Tremblay, et al. Role of deep abdominal fat in the association between regional adipose tissue distribution and glucose tolerance in obese women. *Diabetes* 1989;38:304–09.

Okosun, I. S., K. M. Chandra, S. Choi, et al. 2001. Hypertension and type 2 diabetes comorbidity in adults in the United States: Risk of overall and regional adiposity. *Obesity Res* 2001;9(1):1–9.

Tankó, L. B., Y. Z. Bagger, P. Alexandersen, et al. Peripheral adiposity exhibits an independent dominant antiatherogenic effect in elderly women. *Circulation* 2003;107(12):1626–31.

Chapter 2

Albu, J. B., L. Murphy, D. H. Frager, et al. Visceral fat and race-dependent health risks in obese nondiabetic premenopausal women. *Diabetes* 1997;46(3):456–62.

Barakat, H., R. C. Hickner, J. Privette, et al. Differences in the lipolytic function of adipose tissue preparations from Black American and Caucasian women. *Metabolism* 2002;51(11):1514–18.

Bermudez, O. I., and K. L. Tucker. Total and central obesity among elderly Hispanics and the association with type 2 diabetes. *Obes Res* 2001;9(8):443–51.

Després, J. P., I. Lemieux, and D. Prud'homme. Treatment of obesity: Need to focus on high risk abdominally obese patients. *BMJ* 2001;322:716–20.

Folsom, A. R., L. H. Kushi, K. E. Anderson, et al. Associations of general and abdominal obesity with multiple health outcomes in older women. *Arch Intern Med* 2000;160:2117–2128.

Fontaine, K. R., D. T. Redden, C. Wang, et al. Years of life lost due to obesity. *JAMA* 2003;289(2):187–93.

Han, T. S., P. Richmond, A. Avenell, and M. E. Lean. Waist circumference reduction and cardiovascular benefits during weight loss in women. *Int J Obes Relat Metab Disord* 1997;21(2):127–34.

Hill, J. O. What to do about the metabolic syndrome. *Arch Intern Med* 2003;163:395–97.

Janssen, I., P. T. Katzmarzyk, and R. Ross. Body mass index, waist circumference, and health risk: Evidence in support of current National Institutes of Health guidelines. *Arch Intern Med* 2002;162:2074–79.

Kanaley, J. A., G. Giannoupoulou, G. Tillapaugh-Fay, et al. Racial differences in subcutaneous and visceral fat distribution in postmenopausal black and white women. *Metabolism* 2003;52(3):186–91.

Kurpad, S. S., H. Tandon, and K. Srinivasan. Waist circumference correlates better with body mass index than waist-to-hip ratio in Asian Indians. *Natl Med J India* 2003;16:189–92.

Lean, M. E. J., T. S. Han, and C. E. Morrison. Waist circumference as a measure for indicating need for weight management. *BMJ* 1995;311:158–61.

Lean, M. E., T. S. Han, and J. C. Seidell. Impairment of health and quality of life in people with large waist circumference. *Lancet* 1998;351(9106):853–56.

Lear, S. A., M. M. Chen, J. J. Frohlich, and C. L. Birmingham. The relationship between waist circumference and metabolic risk factors: Cohorts of European and Chinese descent. *Metabolism* 2002;51(11):1427–32.

Lear, S. A., M. M. Chen, C. L. Birmingham, and J. J. Frohlich. The relationship between simple anthropometric indices and C-reactive protein: Ethnic and gender differences. *Metabolism* 2003;52(12):1542–46.

Lissner, L., C. Björkelund, B. L. Heitmann, et al. Larger hip circumference independently predicts health and longevity in a Swedish female cohort. *Obes Res* 2001;9(10):644–46.

Okosun, I. S., Y. Liao, C. N. Rotimi, et al. Abdominal adiposity and clustering of multiple metabolic syndrome in white, black, and Hispanic Americans. *Ann Epidemiol* 2000;10(5):263–270.

Rexrode, K. M., V. J. Carey, C. H. Hennekens, et al. Abdominal adiposity and coronary heart disease in women. *JAMA* 1998;280(21):1843–1848.

Rönnemaa, T., M. Koskenvuo, J. Marniemi, et al. Glucose metabolism in identical twins discordant for obesity: The critical role of visceral fat. *J Clin Endocrinol Metab* 1997;82:383–87.

Sanchez-Castillo, C. P., O. Velazquez-Monroy, A. Berber, et al. Anthropometric cutoff points for predicting chronic diseases in the Mexican National Health Survey 2000. *Obes Res* 2003;11(3):442–51.

Smith, S. R., and J. J. Zachwieja. Visceral adipose tissue: A critical review of intervention strategies. *Int J Obes Relat Metab Disord* 1999;23(4):329–35.

Snehalatha, C., V. Viswanathan, and A. Ramachandran. Cutoff values for normal anthropometric variables in Asian Indian adults. *Diabetes Care* 2003;26(5):1380–84.

Tankó, L. B., Y. Z. Bagger, P. Alexandersen, et al. Central and peripheral fat mass have contrasting effect on the progression of aortic calcification in postmenopausal women. *Eur Heart J* 2003;24(16):1531–37.

Terry, R. B., M. L. Stefanick, W. L. Haskell, and P. D. Wood. Contributions of regional adipose tissue depots to plasma lipoprotein concentrations in overweight men and women: Possible protective effects of thigh fat. *Metabolism* 1991;40(7):733–40.

van Noord, P. A., J. C. Seidell, I. den Tonkelaar, et al. The relationship between fat distribution and some chronic diseases in 11,825 women participating in the DOM-project. *Int J Epidemiol* 1990;19(3):564–70.

Wajchenberg, B. L. Subcutaneous and visceral adipose tissue: Their relation to the metabolic syndrome. *Endocrine Rev* 2000;21(6):697–738.

World Health Organization. September 3, 2003. Controlling the global obesity epidemic. Website:www.who.int/nut/obs.htm.

Zhu, S., Z. Wang, S. Heshka, et al. Waist circumference and obesity-associated risk factors among whites in the third National Health and Nutrition Examination Survey: Clinical action thresholds. *Am J Clin Nutr* 2002;76(4):743–49.

Bjorkelund, C., L. Lissner, S. Andersson, et al. Reproductive history in relation to relative weight and fat distribution. *Int J Obes Relat Metab Disord* 1996;20(3):213–19.

Booth, M. L., T. Chey, and M. Wake, et al. Change in the prevalence of overweight and obesity among young Australians, 1969–1997. *Am J Clin Nutr* 2003;77(1):29–36.

Bowman, S. A., S. L. Gortmaker, C. B. Ebbeling, et al. Effects of fast-food consumption on energy intake and diet quality among children in a national household survey. *Pediatrics* 2004;113(1):112–18.

Giammattei, J., G. Blix, H. H. Marshak, et al. Television watching and soft drink consumption: Associations with obesity in 11- to 13-year-old schoolchildren. *Arch Pediatr Adolesc Med* 2003;157(9):882–86.

Harris, H. E., G. T. Ellison, L. M. Richter, et al. Are overweight women at increased risk of obesity following pregnancy? *Br J Nutr* 1998;79(6):489–94.

Kaur, H., W. S. Choi, M. S. Mayo, and K. J. Harris. Duration of television watching is associated with increased body mass index. *J Pediatr* 2003;143(4):506–11.

Landon, M. B., K. Osei, and M. Platt, et al. The differential effects of body fat distribution on insulin and glucose metabolism during pregnancy. *Am J Obstet Gynecol* 1994;171(4):875–84.

Linne, Y., L. Dye, B. Barkeling, and S. Rossner. Weight development over time in parous women – the SPAWN study – 15 years follow-up. *Int J Obes Relat Metab Disord* 2003;27(12):1516–22.

Linne, Y., and S. Rossner. Interrelationships between weight development and weight retention in subsequent pregnancies: The SPAWN study. *Acta Obstet Gynecol Scand* 2003;82(4):318–25.

Lissau, I., M. D. Overpeck, W. J. Ruan, et al. Body mass index and overweight in adolescents in 13 European countries, Israel, and the United States. *Arch Pediatr Adolesc Med* 2004;158(1):27–33.

McCarthy, H. D., S. M. Ellis, and T. J. Cole. Central overweight and obesity in British youth aged 11–16 years: Cross sectional surveys of waist circumference. *BMJ* 2003;326(7390):624.

Pascot, A., S. Lemieux, I. Lemieux, et al. Age-related increase in visceral adipose tissue and body fat and the metabolic risk profile of premenopausal women. *Diabetes Care* 1999;22(9):1471–78.

Pi-Sunyer, F. X. Obesity. In: Shils, M. E., J. A. Olson, M. Shike, and A. C. Ross, eds. *Modern Nutrition in Health and Disease,* 9th edition. Philadelphia, PA: Williams & Wilkins, 1999;1395–1408.

Robinson, T. N. Reducing children's television viewing to prevent obesity. *JAMA* 1999;282(16):1561–67.

Rodrigues, M. L., and T. H. Da Costa. Association of the maternal experience and changes in adiposity measured by BMI, waist:hip ratio and per centage body fat in urban Brazilian women. *Br J Nutr* 2001;85(1):107–14.

Sattar, N., P. Clark, and A. Holmes, et al. Antenatal waist circumference and hypertension risk. *Obstet Gynecol* 2001;97(2):268–71.

Scholl, T. O., and X. Chen. Insulin and the 'thrifty' woman: The influence of insulin during pregnancy on gestational weight gain and postpartum weight retention. *Matern Child Health J* 2002;6(4):255–61.

Schwimmer, J. B., T. M. Burwinkle, and J. W. Varni. Health-related quality of life of severely obese children and adolescents. *JAMA* 2003;289(14):1813–19.

Sidebottom, A. C., J. E. Brown, and D. R. Jacobs Jr. Pregnancy-related changes in body fat. *Eur J Obstet Gynecol Reprod Biol* 2001;94(2):216–23.

Smith, D. E., C. E. Lewis, J. L. Caveny, et al. Longitudinal changes in adiposity associated with pregnancy: The CARDIA study. Coronary Artery Risk Development in Young Adults study. *JAMA* 1994;271(22):1747–51.

Soltani, H., and R. B. Fraser. A longitudinal study of maternal anthropometric changes in normal weight, overweight and obese women during pregnancy and postpartum. *Br J Nutr* 2000;84:95–101.

Sowers, M. F., M. Crutchfield, M. L. Jannausch, and M. Russell-Aulet. Longitudinal changes in body composition in women approaching the midlife. *Ann Hum Biol* 1996;23(3):253–65.

Storey, M. L., R. A. Forshee, A. R. Weaver, and W. R. Sansalone. Demographic and lifestyle factors associated with body mass index among children and adolescents. *Int J Food Sci Nutr* 2003;54(6):491–503.

Svendsen, O. L., C. Hassager, and C. Christiansen. Age- and menopause-associated variation in body composition and fat distribution in healthy women as measured by dual-energy x-ray absorptiometry. *Metabolism* 1995;44(3):369–73.

Tankó, L. B. What trends can be observed in peripheral overweight among upcoming generation of women? Comment in response to McCarthy, et al. 2003. Internet: http://bmj.bmjjournals.com/cgi/eletters/326/7390/624. Accessed: January 6, 2004.

Toth, M. J., A. Tchernof, C. K. Sites, and E. T. Poehlman. Menopause-related changes in body fat distribution. *Ann NY Acad Sci* 2000;904:502–06.

Tremollieres, F. A., J. M. Pouilles, and C. A. Ribot. Relative influence of age and menopause on total and regional body composition changes in postmenopausal women. *Am J Obstet Gynecol* 1996;175(6):1594–1600.

Wolfe, W. S., J. Sobal, C. M. Olson, et al. Parity-associated weight gain and its modification by sociodemographic and behavioral factors: A prospective analysis in US women. *Int J Obes Relat Metab Disord* 1997;21(9):802–10.

Yamamoto, S., T. Douchi, N. Yoshimitsu, et al. Waist to hip circumference ratio as a significant predictor of pre-eclampsia, irrespective of overall adiposity. *J Obstet Gynaecol Res* 2001;27(1):27–31.

Zhang, S., A. R. Folsom, J. M. Flack, and K. Liu. Body fat distribution before pregnancy and gestational diabetes: Findings from coronary artery risk development in young adults (CARDIA) study. *BMJ* 1995;311(7013):1139–40.

Chapter 4

Albertazzi, P., and D. W. Purdie. The nature and utility of the phytooestrogens: A review of the evidence. *Maturitas* 2002;42:173–85.

American College of Obstetricians and Gynecologists Committee on Practice Bulletins – Gynecology. ACOG Practice Bulletin. Clinical management guidelines for obstetrician-gynecologists. Use of botanicals for management of menopausal symptoms. *Obstet Gynecol* 2001;97(6):suppl 1–11.

Barinas-Mitchell, E., M. Cushman, E. N. Meilahn, et al. Serum levels of C-reactive protein are associated with obesity, weight gain, and hormone replacement therapy in healthy postmenopausal women. *Am J Epidemiol* 2001;153(11):1094–1101.

Burger, H. Hormone replacement therapy in the post-Women's Health Initiative era. Report on a meeting held in Funchal, Madeira. February 24–25, 2003. *Climacteric* 2003;6 Suppl 1:11–36.

Douchi, T., R. Kuwahata, S. Yamamoto, et al. Relationship of upper body obesity to menstrual disorders. *Acta Obstet Gynecol Scand* 2002;81:147–50.

Faure, E. D., P. Chantre, and P. Mares. Effects of a standardized soy extract on hot flushes: A multicenter, double-blind, randomized, placebo-controlled study. *Menopause* 2002;9(5):329–34.

Hirata, J. D., L. M. Swiersz, B. Zell, et al. Does dong quai have oestrogenic effects in postmenopausal women? A double-blind, placebo-controlled trial. *Fertil Steril* 1997;68(6):981–86.

Hollmann, M., B. Runnebaum, and I. Gerhard. Impact of waist-hip-ratio and body-mass-index on hormonal and metabolic parameters in young, obese women. *Int J Obes Relat Metab Disord* 1997;21(6):476–83.

Jenkins, D. J., C. W. Kendall, C. J. Jackson, et al. Effects of high- and low-isoflavone soyfoods on blood lipids, oxidized LDL, homocysteine, and blood pressure in hyperlipidemic men and women. *Am J Clin Nutr* 2002;76(2):365–72.

Kang, H. J., R. Ansbacher, and M. M. Hammoud. Use of alternative and complementary medicine in menopause. *Int J Gynecol Obstet* 2002;79:195–207.

Kirschner, M. A., E. Samojlik, M. Drejka, et al. Androgen-oestrogen metabolism in women with upper body versus lower body obesity. *J Clin Enocrinol Metab* 1990;70(2):473–79.

Kligler, B. Black cohosh. *Am Fam Physician* 2003;68(1):114–16.

Komesaroff, P. A., C. V. Black, V. Cable, and K. Sudhir. Effects of wild yam extract on menopausal symptoms, lipids and sex hormones in healthy menopausal women. *Climacteric* 2001;4(2):144–150.

Kronenberg, F., and A. Fugh-Berman. Complementary and alternative medicine for menopausal symptoms: A review of randomized, controlled trials. *Ann Intern Med* 2002;137(10):805–13.

Lucks, B. C. *Vitex agnus castus* essential oil and menopausal balance. *Complement Ther Nurs Midwif* 2003;9:157–60.

Messina, M., and C. Hughes. Efficacy of soyfoods and soybean isoflavone supplements for alleviating menopausal symptoms is positively related to initial hot flush frequency. *J Med Food* 2003;6(1):1–11.

North American Menopause Society. Treatment of menopause-associated vasomotor symptoms: Position statement of The North American Menopause Society. *Menopause* 2004;11(1):11–33.

Perry, A. C., M. Allison, E. B. Applegate, et al. The relationship between fat distribution and coronary risk factors in sedentary postmenopausal women on and off hormone replacement therapy. *Obes Res* 1998;6(1):40–46.

Ryan, A. S., B. J. Nicklas, and D. M. Berman. Hormone replacement therapy, insulin sensitivity, and abdominal obesity in postmenopausal women. *Diabetes Care* 2002;25(1):127–33.

Shanafelt, T. D., D. L. Barton, A. A. Adjei, and C. L. Loprinzi. Pathophysiology and treatment of hot flashes. *Mayo Clin Proc* 2002;77(11):1207–18.

Stearns, V., K. L. Beebe, M. Iyengar, and E. Dube. Paroxetine controlled release in the treatment of menopausal hot flashes: A randomized controlled trial. *JAMA* 2003;289(21):2827–34.

Tchernof, A., E. T. Poehlman, and J. P. Despres. Body fat distribution, the menopause transition, and hormone replacement therapy. *Diabetes Metab* 2000;26(1):12–20.

Teschke, R., W. Gaus, and D. Loew. Kava extracts: Safety and risks including rare hepatotoxicity. *Phytomedicine* 2003;10(5):440–46.

Tham, D. M., C. D. Gardner, and W. L. Haskell. Clinical Review 97. Potential health benefits of dietary phytooestrogens: A review of the clinical, epidemiological, and mechanistic evidence. *J Clin Endocrinol Metab* 1998;83(7):2223–35.

Tice, J. A., B. Ettinger, K. Ensrud, et al. Phytooestrogen supplements for the treatment of hot flashes: The Isoflavone Clover Extract (ICE) study: A randomized controlled trial. *JAMA* 2003;290(2):207–14.

Wren, B. G., S. M. Champion, K. Willetts, et al. Transdermal progesterone and its effect on vasomotor symptoms, blood lipid levels, bone metabolic markers, moods, and quality of life for postmenopausal women. *Menopause* 2003;10(1):13–18.

Writing Group for the Women's Health Initiative Investigators. Risks and benefits of oestrogen plus progestin in healthy postmenopausal women. *JAMA* 2002;288(3):321–33.

Yamamoto, S., T. Sobue, M. Kobayashi, et al. Soy, isoflavones, and breast cancer risk in Japan. *J Natl Cancer Inst* 2003;95(12):906–13.

Chapter 5

Abate, N., and M. Chandalia. Ethnicity and type 2 diabetes: Focus on Asian Indians. *J Diabetes Compl* 2001;15:320–27.

Astrup, A., and N. Finer. Redefining type 2 diabetes: 'Diabesity' or 'obesity dependent diabetes mellitus'? *Obesity Rev* 2000;1(2):57–59.

Bonds, D. E., D. J. Zaccaro, A. J. Karter, et al. Ethnic and racial differences in diabetes care. *Diabetes Care* 2003;26(4):1040–46.

Brochu, M., A. Tchernof, I. J. Dionne, et al. What are the physical characteristics associated with a normal metabolic profile despite a high level of obesity in postmenopausal women? *J Clin Endocrinol Metab* 2001;86:1020–25.

Carey, V. J., E. E. Walters, G. A. Colditz, et al. Body fat distribution and risk of non-insulin-dependent diabetes mellitus in women. The Nurses' Health Study. *Am J Epidemiol* 1997;145(7):614–19.

Centers for Disease Control and Prevention. Diabetes prevalence among

American Indians and Alaska Natives and the overall population – United States, 1994–2002. *MMWR Morb Mortal Wkly Rpt* 2003;52(30):702–04.

Clark, C. M., J. E. Fradkin, R. G. Hiss, et al. Promoting early diagnosis and treatment of type 2 diabetes. The National Diabetes Education Program. *JAMA* 2000;284(3):363–64.

Collins, T. C., M. Johnson, W. Henderson, et al. Lower extremity non-traumatic amputation among veterans with peripheral arterial disease: Is race an independent factor? *Med Care* 2002;40(1 suppl):I106–16.

Dalton, M., A. J. Cameron, P. Z. Zimmet, et al. Waist circumference, waist-hip ratio and body mass index and their correlation with cardiovascular disease risk factors in Australian adults. *J Intern Med* 2003;254:555–63.

Diabetes Prevention Program Study Group. Reduction in the incidence of type 2 diabetes with lifestyle intervention or metformin. *N Engl J Med* 2002;346:393–403.

Dvorak, R. V., W. F. DeNino, P. A. Ades, and E. T. Poehlman. Phenotypic characteristics associated with insulin resistance in metabolically obese but normal-weight young women. *Diabetes* 1999;48:2210–14.

Gary, T. L., K. M. Narayan, E. W. Gregg, et al. Racial/ethnic differences in the healthcare experience (coverage, utilization, and satisfaction) of US adults with diabetes. *Ethn Dis* 2003;13(1):47–54.

Gastaldelli, A., Y. Miyazaki, M. Pettiti, et al. Metabolic effects of visceral fat accumulation in type 2 diabetes. *J Clin Endocrinol Metab* 2002;87(11):5098–5103.

Glueck, C. J., R. Papanna, P. Wang, et al. Incidence and treatment of metabolic syndrome in newly referred women with confirmed polycystic ovarian syndrome. *Metabolism* 2003;52:908–15.

Harris, M. I., K. M. Flegal, C. C. Cowie, et al. Prevalence of diabetes, impaired fasting glucose, and impaired glucose tolerance in U.S. adults. The third National Health and Nutrition Examination Survey, 1988–1994. *Diabetes Care* 1998;21(4):518–24.

Hill, J. O., J. Hauptman, J. W. Anderson, et al. Orlistat, a lipase inhibitor, for weight maintenance after conventional dieting: A 1-y study. *Am J Clin Nutr* 1999;69:1108–16.

Hollander, P. A., S. C. Elbein, I. B. Hirsch, et al. Role of orlistat in the treatment of obese patients with type 2 diabetes. *Diabetes Care* 1998;21(8):1288–94.

Hu, F. B., J. E. Manson, M. J. Stampfer, et al. Diet, lifestyle, and the risk of type 2 diabetes mellitus in women. *N Engl J Med* 2001;345(11):790–97.

Jee, S. H., S. Y. Lee, C. M. Nam, et al. Effect of smoking on the paradox of high waist-to-hip ratio and low body mass index. *Obes Res* 2002;10(9):891–95.

Kahn, H. S., and R. Valdez. Metabolic risks identified by the combination of enlarged waist and elevated triacylglycerol concentration. *Am J Clin Nutr* 2003;78(5):928–34.

Karter, A. J., A. Ferrara, J. Y. Liu, et al. Ethnic disparities in diabetic complications in an insured population. *JAMA* 2002;287(19):2519–27.

Konen, J. C., J. H. Summerson, R. A. Bell, and L. G. Curtis. Racial differences in symptoms and complications in adults with type 2 diabetes mellitus. *Ethn Health* 1999;4(1–2):39–49.

Lemieux, I., A. Pascot, C. Couillard, et al. Hypertriglyceridemic waist: A marker of the atherogenic metabolic triad (hyperinsulinemia; hyperapoli-poprotein B; small, dense LDL) in men? *Circulation* 2000;102:179–84.

Matsuzawa, Y., I. Shimomura, T. Nakamura, et al. Pathophysiology and pathogenesis of visceral fat obesity. *Obes Res* 1995;3(suppl 2):187S–194S.

Meacham, L. R., H. Abdul-Latif, K. Sullivan, and F. L. Culler. Predictors of change in insulin sensitivity during glucocorticoids treatment. *Horm Metab Res* 1997;29(4):172–75.

Pasquali, R., A. Gambineri, B. Anconetani, et al. The natural history of the metabolic syndrome in young women with the polycystic ovary syndrome and the effect of long-term ooestrogen-progestagen treatment. *Clin Endocrinol* 1999;50:517–27.

Perry, C. G., A. Spiers, S. J. Cleland, et al. Glucocorticoids and insulin sensitivity: Dissociation of insulin's metabolic and vascular actions. *J Clin Endocrinol Metab* 2003;88(12):6008–14.

Rimm, E. B., J. Chan, M. J. Stampfer, et al. Prospective study of cigarette smoking, alcohol use, and the risk of diabetes in men. *BMJ* 1995;310(6979):555–59.

Rimm, E. B., J. E. Manson, M. J. Stampfer, et al. Cigarette smoking and the risk of diabetes in women. *Am J Public Health* 1993;83(2):211–14.

Shaw, J. E., and D. J. Chisholm. 1. Epidemiology and prevention of type 2 diabetes and the metabolic syndrome. *Med J Aust* 2003;179(7):379–83.

Snijder, M. B., J. M. Dekker, M. Visser, et al. Associations of hip and thigh circumferences independent of waist circumference with the incidence of type 2 diabetes: The Hoorn Study. *Am J Clin Nutr* 2003;77(5):1192–97.

Spiegel, K., R. Leproult, and E. Van Cauter. Impact of sleep debt on metabolic and endocrine function. *Lancet* 1999;354(9188):1435–39.

Stoney, R. M., K. Z. Walker, J. D. Best, et al. Do postmenopausal women with

NIDDM have a reduced capacity to deposit and conserve lower-body fat? *Diabetes Care* 1998;21(5):828–30.

Summerson, J. H., R. A. Bell, J. C. Konen, and J. G. Spangler. Differential impact of cardiovascular disease (CVD) risk factor clustering on CVD and renal disease among African-American and white patients with type 2 diabetes mellitus. *Ethn Dis* 2002;12(4):530–34.

Tuomilehto, J., J. Lindström, J. G. Eriksson, et al. Prevention of type 2 diabetes mellitus by changes in lifestyle among subjects with impaired glucose tolerance. *N Engl J Med* 2001;344:1343–50.

Wollin, S. D., and P. J. Jones. Alcohol, red wine and cardiovascular disease. *J Nutr* 2001;131:1401–04.

Young, B. A., C. Maynard, and E. J. Boyko. Racial differences in diabetic neuropathy, cardiovascular disease, and mortality in a national population of veterans. *Diabetes Care* 2003;26(8):2392–99.

Zimmet, P., K. G. M. M. Alberti, and J. Shaw. Global and societal implications of the diabetes epidemic. *Nature* 2001;414:782–87.

Chapter 6

Ciubotaru, I., Y. S. Lee, and R. C. Wander. Dietary fish oil decreases C-reactive protein, interleukin-6, and triacylglycerol to HDL-cholesterol ratio in postmenopausal women on HRT. *J Nutr Biochem* 2003;14(9):513–21.

Cole, S. R., I. Kawachi, S. Liu, et al. Time urgency and risk of non-fatal myocardial infarction. *Int J Epidemiol* 2001;30(2):363–69.

Dallongeville, J., J. Yarnell, P. Ducimetiere, et al. Fish consumption is associated with lower heart rates. *Circulation* 2003;108(7):820–25.

Gasteyger, C., and A. Tremblay. Metabolic impact of body fat distribution. *J Endocrinol Invest* 2002;25(10):876–83.

Hu, D., J. Hannah, R. S. Gray, et al. Effects of obesity and body fat distribution on lipids and lipoproteins in nondiabetic American Indians: The Strong Heart Study. *Obes Res* 2000;8(6):411–21.

Kanety, H., R. Feinstein, M. Z. Papa, et al. Tumor necrosis factor alpha-induced phosphorylation of insulin receptor substrate-1 (IRS-1). Possible mechanism for suppression of insulin-stimulated tyrosine phosphorylation of IRS-1. *J Biol Chem* 1995;270(40):23780–84.

Lemieux, I., A. Paascot, D. Prud'homme, et al. Elevated C-reactive protein. Another component of the atherothrombotic profile of abdominal obesity. *Arterioscler Thromb Vasc Biol* 2001;21:961–67.

Lyon, C. J., R. E. Law, and W. A. Hsueh. Minireview: Adiposity, inflammation, and atherogenesis. *Endocrinology* 2003;144(6):2195–2200.

Nesto, R. W. The relation of insulin resistance syndromes to risk of cardiovascular disease. *Rev Cardiovasc Med* 2003;4(suppl6):S11–S18.

Rexrode, K. M., V. J. Carey, C. H. Hennekens, et al. Abdominal adiposity and coronary heart disease in women. *JAMA* 1998;280(21):1843–48.

Rexrode, K. M., A. Pradhan, J. E. Manson, et al. Relationship of total and abdominal adiposity with CRP and IL-6 in women. *Ann Epidemiol* 2003;13(10):674–82.

Rich-Edwards, J. W., J. E. Manson, C. H. Hennekens, and J. E. Buring. The primary prevention of coronary disease in women. *New Engl J Med* 1995;332(26):1758–66.

Ridker, P. M. High-sensitivity C-reactive protein and cardiovascular risk: Rationale for screening and primary prevention. *Am J Cardiol* 2003;92(suppl 2):17K–22K.

Ridker, P. M., N. Rifai, L. Rose, et al. Comparison of C-reactive protein and low-density lipoprotein cholesterol levels in the prediction of first cardiovascular events. *N Engl J Med* 2002;347(20):1557–65.

Solomon, C. G., F. B. Hu, A. Dunaif, et al. Menstrual cycle irregularity and risk for future cardiovascular disease. *J Clin Endocrinol Metab* 2002;87(5):2013–17.

Suk, S. H., R. L. Sacco, B. Boden-Albala, et al. Abdominal obesity and risk of ischemic stroke: The Northern Manhattan Stroke Study. *Stroke* 2003;34(7):1586–92.

Terry, R. B., M. L. Stefanick, W. L. Haskell, and P. D. Wood. Contributions of regional adipose tissue depots to plasma lipoprotein concentrations in overweight men and women: Possible protective effects of thigh fat. *Metabolism* 1991;40(7):733–40.

Tice, J. A., W. Borwner, R. P. Tracy, and S. R. Cummings. The relation of C-reactive protein levels to total and cardiovascular mortality in older U.S. women. *Am J Med* 2003;114(3):199–205.

Van Pelt, R. E., E. M. Evans, K. B. Schechtman, et al. Contributions of total and regional fat mass to risk for cardiovascular disease in older women. *Am J Physiol Endocrinol Metab* 2002;282(5):E1023–E1028.

Welborn, T. A., S. S. Dhaliwal, and S. A. Bennett. Waist-hip ratio is the dominant risk factor predicting cardiovascular death in Australia. *Med J Aust* 2003;179(11–12):580–85.

Williams, M. J., G. R. Hunter, T. Kekes-Szabo, et al. Regional fat distribution in women and risk of cardiovascular disease. *Am J Clin Nutr* 1997;65(3):855–60.

Wingo, P. A., E. E. Calle, and A. McTiernan. How does breast cancer mortality compare with that of other cancers and selected cardiovascular diseases at different ages in U.S. women? *J Womens Health Gend Based Med* 2000;9(9):999–1006.

Ziccardi, P., F. Nappo, G. Giugliano, et al. Reduction of inflammatory cytokine concentrations and improvement of endothelial functions in obese women after weight loss over one year. *Circulation* 2002;105(7):804–09.

Chapter 7

Ballard-Barbash, R., and C. A. Swanson. Body weight: Estimation of risk for breast and endometrial cancers. *Am J Clin Nutr* 1996;63(3 suppl): 437S–441S.

Barnett, J. B. The relationship between obesity and breast cancer risk and mortality. *Nutr Rev* 2003;61(2):73–76.

Connolly, B. S., C. Barnett, K. N. Vogt, et al. A meta-analysis of published literature on waist-to-hip ratio and risk of breast cancer. *Nutr Cancer* 2002;44(2):127–38.

Davis, S., D. K. Mirick, and R. G. Stevens. Night shift work, light at night, and risk of breast cancer. *J Natl Cancer Inst* 2001;93(20):1557–62.

Friedenreich, C. M., K. S. Courneya, and H. E. Bryant. Case-control study of anthropometric measures and breast cancer risk. *Int J Cancer* 2002;99(3):445–52.

Huang, Z., S. E. Hankinson, G. A. Colditz, et al. Dual effects of weight and weight gain on breast cancer risk. *JAMA* 1997;278(17):1407–11.

Huang, Z., W. C. Willett, G. A. Colditz, et al. Waist circumference, waist:hip ratio, and risk of breast cancer in the Nurses' Health Study. *Am J Epidemiol* 1999;150(12):1316–24.

Iemura, A., T. Douchi, S. Yamamoto, et al. Body fat distribution as a risk factor of endometrial cancer. *J Obstet Gynaecol Res* 2000;26(6):421–25.

Key, T. J., N. E. Allen, E. A. Spencer, and R. C. Travis. Nutrition and breast cancer. *Breast* 2003;12(6):412–16.

Key, T. J., P. N. Appleby, G. K. Reeves, et al. Body mass index, serum sex hormones, and breast cancer risk in postmenopausal women. *J Natl Cancer Inst* 2003;95(16):1218–26.

Kropp, S., and J. Chang-Claude. Active and passive smoking and risk of breast cancer by age 50 years among German women. *Am J Epidemiol* 2002;156:616–26.

Morimoto, L. M., E. White, Z. Chen, et al. Obesity, body size, and risk of postmenopausal breast cancer: The Women's Health Initiative (United States). *Cancer Causes Control* 2002;13(8):741–51.

Olson, J. E., P. Yang, K. Schmitz, et al. Differential association of body mass index and fat distribution with three major histologic types of lung cancer: Evidence from a cohort of older women. *Am J Epidemiol* 2002;156:606–15.

Parker, E. D., and A. R. Folsom. Intentional weight loss and incidence of obesity-related cancers: The Iowa Women's Health study. *Int J Obes Relat Metab Disord* 2003;27(12):1447–52.

Rossouw, J. E., G. L. Anderson, R. L. Prentice, et al. Risks and benefits of oestrogen plus progestin in healthy postmenopausal women: Principal results from the Women's Health Initiative randomized controlled trial. *JAMA* 2002;288(3):321–33.

Sephton, S., and D. Spiegel. Circadian disruption in cancer: A neuro-endocrine-immune pathway from stress to disease? *Brain Behav Immun* 2003;17(5):321–28.

Shimokata, H., D. C. Muller, and R. Andres. Studies in the distribution of body fat. III. Effects of cigarette smoking. *JAMA* 1989;261(8):1169–73.

Sonnenschein, E., P. Toniolo, M. B. Terry, et al. Body fat distribution and obesity in pre- and postmenopausal breast cancer. *Int J Epidemiol* 1999;28:1026–31.

Swanson, C. A., N. Potischman, G. D. Wilbanks, et al. Relation of endometrial cancer risk to past and contemporary body size and body fat distribution. *Cancer Epidemiol Biomarkers Prev* 1993;2(4):321–27.

Chapter 8

Angus, R. M., P. N. Sambrook, N. A. Pocock, and J. A. Eisman. Dietary intake and bone mineral density. *Bone Miner* 1988;4(3):265–77.

Blain, H., A. Vuillemin, A. Teissier, et al. Influence of muscle strength and body weight and composition on regional bone mineral density in healthy women aged 60 years and over. *Gerontology* 2001;47(4):207–12.

Conlisk, A. J., and D. A. Galuska. Is caffeine associated with bone mineral density in young adult women? *Prev Med* 2000;31(5):562–68.

Cooper, C., E. J. Atkinson, H. W. Wahner, et al. Is caffeine consumption a risk factor for osteoporosis? *J Bone Miner Res* 1992;7(4):465–71.

Douchi, T., T. Oki, S. Nakamura, et al. The effect of body composition on bone density in pre- and postmenopausal women. *Maturitas* 1997;27:55–60.

Douchi, T., S. Yamamoto, T. Oki, et al. Relationship between body fat distribution and bone mineral density in premenopausal Japanese women. *Obstet Gynecol* 2000;95(5):722–25.

Earnshaw, S. A., A. Worley, and D. J. Hosking. Current diet does not relate to bone mineral density after the menopause: The Nottingham Early Postmenopausal Intervention Cohort (EPIC) study group. *Br J Nutr* 1997;78(1):65–72.

Feskanich, D., W. C. Willett, M. J. Stampfer, and G. A. Colditz. A prospective study of thiazide use and fractures in women. *Osteoporos Int* 1997;7(1):79–84.

Heaney, R. P. Effects of caffeine on bone and the calcium economy. *Food Chem Toxicol* 2002;40(9):1263–70.

Heaney, R. P., and K. Rafferty. Carbonated beverages and urinary calcium excretion. *Am J Clin Nutr* 2001;74(3):343–47.

Jeffcoat, M. K., and C. H. Chesnut III. Systemic osteoporosis and oral bone loss: Evidence shows increased risk factors. *J Am Dent Assoc* 1993;124(11):49–56.

Kirchengast, S., B. Peterson, G. Hauser, and W. Knogler. Bone composition characteristics are associated with the bone density of the proximal femur end in middle- and old-aged women and men. *Maturitas* 2001;39:133–45.

Layne, J. E., and M. E. Nelson. The effects of resistance training on bone density: A review. *Med Sci Sports Exerc* 1999;31(1):25–30.

L'Hermitte, F., A. Behar, J. Pariès, et al. Impairment of lymphatic function in women with gynoid adiposity and swelling syndrome. *Metabolism* 2003;52(7):805–09.

Lloyd, T., N. Rollings, D. F. Eggli, et al. Dietary caffeine intake and bone status of postmenopausal women. *Am J Clin Nutr* 1997;65(5):1826–30.

Macdonald, H. M., S. A. New, M. H. Golden, et al. Nutritional associations with bone loss during the menopausal transition: Evidence of a beneficial effect of calcium, alcohol, and fruit and vegetable nutrients and of a detrimental effect of fatty acids. *Am J Clin Nutr* 2004;79(1):155–65.

Matsuo, T., T. Douchi, M. Nakae, et al. Relationship of upper body fat distribution to higher regional lean mass and bone mineral density. *J Bone Miner Metab* 2003;21:179–83.

Mohammad, A. R., D. A. Hooper, S. G. Vermilyea, et al. An investigation of the relationship between systemic bone density and clinical periodontal status in post-menopausal Asian-American women. *Int Dent J* 2003;53(3):121–25.

Murillo-Uribe, A., S. Carranza-Lira, N. Martinez-Trejo, and J. Santos-Gonzalez. Influence of weight and body fat distribution on bone density in postmenopausal women. *Int J Fertil Womens Med* 2000;45(3):225–31.

Nelson, M. E., M. A. Fiatarone, C. M. Morganti, et al. Effects of high-intensity strength training on multiple risk factors for osteoporotic fractures: A randomized controlled trial. *JAMA* 1994;272(24):1909–1914.

Notelovitz, M. Androgen effects on bone and muscle. *Fertil Steril* 2002;77(suppl 4):S34–S41.

Ortego-Centeno, N., M. Munoz-Torres, J. Hernandez-Quero, et al. Bone mineral density, sex steroids, and mineral metabolism in premenopausal smokers. *Calcif Tissue Int* 1994;55(6):403–07.

Seidell, J. C., J. C. Bakx, E. De Boer, et al. Fat distribution of overweight persons in relation to morbidity and subjective health. *Int J Obes* 1985;9(5):363–74.

Smith, S., J. Swain, E. M. Brown, et al. A preliminary report of the short-term effect of carbonated beverage consumption on calcium metabolism in normal women. *Arch Intern Med* 1989;149(11):2517–19.

Turner, L. W., M. A. Bass, L. Ting, and B. Brown. Influence of yard work and weight training on bone mineral density among older U.S. women. *J Women Aging* 2002;14(3–4):139–48.

van Noord, P. A., J. C. Seidell, I. den Tonkelaar, et al. The relationship between fat distribution and some chronic diseases in 11,825 women participating in the DOM-project. *Int J Epidemiol* 1990;19(3):564–70.

Chapter 9

Barden, N., J. M. Reul, and F. Holsboer. Do antidepressants stabilize mood through actions on the hypothalamic-pituitary-adrenocortical system? *Trends Neurosci* 1995;18(1):6–11.

Bell, R. A., J. H. Summerson, J. G. Spangler, and J. C. Konan. Body fat, fat distribution, and psychosocial factors among patients with type 2 diabetes mellitus. *Behav Med* 1998;24(3):138–43.

Berk, L. S., S. A. Tan, W. F. Fry, et al. Neuroendocrine and stress hormone changes during mirthful laughter. *Am J Med Sci* 1989;298(6):390–96.

Björntorp, P. Do stress reactions cause abdominal obesity and comorbidities? *Obes Rev* 2001;2:73–86.

————. Obesity and the adipocyte. *J Endocrinol* 1997;155:193–95.

————. The origins and consequences of obesity. Diabetes. *Ciba Found Symp* 1996;201:68–80.

————. Visceral fat accumulation: The missing link between psychosocial factors and cardiovascular disease? *J Intern Med* 1991;230:195–201.

Björntorp, P., and R. Rosmond. Neuroendocrine abnormalities in visceral obesity. *Int J Obes Relat Metab Disord* 2000;24(suppl 2):S80–S85.

————. Obesity and cortisol. *Nutrition* 2000;16(10):924–36.

Black, P., H. The inflammatory response is an integral part of the stress response: Implications for atherosclerosis, insulin resistance, type II diabetes and metabolic syndrome X. *Brain Behav Immun* 2003;17(5):350–64.

Buckett, W. R., P. C. Thomas, and G. P. Luscombe. The pharmacology of sibutramine hydrochloride (BTS 54 524), a new antidepressant which induces rapid noradrenergic down-regulation. *Prog Neuropsychopharmacol Biol Psychiatry* 1988;12(5):575–84.

Bunker, S. J., D. M. Colquhoun, M. D. Esler, et al. 'Stress' and coronary heart disease: Psychosocial risk factors. *Med J Aust* 2003;178(6):272–76.

Burns, J. W., A. Kubilus, and S. Bruehl. Emotion induction moderates effects of anger management style on acute pain sensitivity. *Pain* 2003;106(1–2):109–18.

Carlson, L. E., M. Speca, K. D. Patel, and E. Goodey. Mindfulness-based stress reduction in relation to quality of life, mood, symptoms of stress and levels of sortisol, dehydroepiandrosterone sulfate (DHEAS) and melatonin in breast and prostate cancer outpatients. *Psychoneuroendocrinol* 2004;28:448–74.

Davis, C., and D. Cerullo. Fat distribution in young women: Associations and interactions with behavioural, physical, and psychological factors. *Psychol Health Med* 1996;1(2):159–67.

Davis, M. C., E. W. Twamley, N. A. Hamilton, and P. D. Swan. Body fat distribution and hemodynamic stress responses in premenopausal obese women: A preliminary study. *Health Psychol* 1999;18(6):625–33.

Demitrack, M. A., and L. J. Rofford. Evidence for and pathophysiologic implications of hypothalamic-pituitary-adrenal axis dysregulation in fibromyalgia and chronic fatigue syndrome. *Ann NY Acad Sci* 1998;840:684–97.

Duclos, M., J. B. Corcuff, N. Etcheverry, et al. Abdominal obesity increases overnight cortisol excretion. *J Endocrinol Invest* 1999;22(6):465–71.

Epel, E., R. Lapidus, B. McEwen, and K. Brownell. Stress may add bite to appetite in women: A laboratory study of stress-induced cortisol and eating behavior. *Psychoneuroendocrinology* 2001;26:37–49.

Epel, E., B. McEwen, T. Seeman, et al. Stress and body shape: Stress-induced cortisol secretion is consistently greater among women with central fat. *Psychosom Med* 2000;62(5):623–32.

Golden, S. H., J. E. Williams, D. E. Ford, et al. Depressive symptoms and the risk of type 2 diabetes: The Atherosclerosis Risk in Communities study. *Diabetes Care* 2004;27(2):429–35.

Griep, E. N., J. W. Boersma, and E. R. de Kloet. Altered reactivity of the hypothalamic-pituitary-adrenal axis in the primary fibromyalgia syndrome. *J Rheumatol* 1993;20(3):469–74.

Harlow, B. L., L. B. Signorello, J. E. Hall, et al. Reproductive correlates of chronic fatigue syndrome. *Am J Med* 1998;105(3A):94S–99S.

Jin, P. Efficacy of Tai Chi, brisk walking, meditation, and reading in reducing mental and emotional stress. *J Psychosom Res* 1992;36(4):361–70.

Kiecolt-Glaser, J. K., K. J. Preacher, R. C. MacCallum, et al. Chronic stress and age-related increases in the proinflammatory cytokine IL-6. *Proc Natl Acad Sci USA* 2003;100(15):9090–95.

Ljung, T., A. C. Ahlberg, G. Holm, et al. Treatment of abdominally obese men with a serotonin reuptake inhibitor: A pilot study. *J Intern Med* 2001;250(3):219–24.

Lloyd, C. E., R. R. Wing, and T. J. Orchard. Waist to hip ratio and psychosocial factors in adults with insulin-dependent diabetes mellitus: The Pittsburgh Epidemiology of Diabetes Complications study. *Metabolism* 1996;45(2):268–72.

Luby, J. L., A. Heffelfinger, C. Mrakotsky, et al. Alterations in stress cortisol reactivity in depressed preschoolers relative to psychiatric and no-disorder comparison groups. *Arch Gen Psychiatry* 2003;60(12):1248–55.

Marin, P., N. Darin, T. Amemiya, et al. Cortisol secretion in relation to body fat distribution in obese premenopausal women. *Metabolism* 1992;41(8):882–86.

McNamara, M. E., D. C. Burnham, C. Smith, and D. L. Carroll. The effects of back massage before diagnostic cardiac catheterization. *Altern Ther Health Med* 2003;9(1):50–57.

Moorkens, G., J. Berwaerts, H. Wynants, and R. Abs. Characterization of pituitary function with emphasis on GH secretion in the chronic fatigue syndrome. *Clin Endocrinol* 2000;53(1):99–106.

Mooy, J. M., H. de Vries, P. A. Grootenhuis, et al. Major stressful life events in relation to prevalence of undetected type 2 diabetes: The Hoorn study. *Diabetes Care* 2000;23(2):197–201.

Murphy, F. C., K. A. Smith, P. J. Cowen, et al. The effects of tryptophan depletion on cognitive and affective processing in healthy volunteers. *Psychopharmacology* (Berl) 2002;163(1):42–53.

Neeck, G., and L. J. Crofford. Neuroendocrine perturbations in fibromyalgia and chronic fatigue syndrome. *Rheum Dis Clin North Am* 2000;26(4):989–1002.

Okugawa, G., K. Omori, J. Suzukawa, et al. Long-term treatment with antidepressants increases glucocorticoids receptor binding and gene expression in cultured rat hippocampal neurons. *J Neuroendocrinol* 1999;11(11):887–95.

Pawlow, L. A., and G. E. Jones. The impact of abbreviated progressive muscle relation on salivary cortisol. *Biol Psychol* 2002;60(1):1–16.

Räikkönen, K., K. A. Matthews, and L. H. Kuller. Anthropometric and psychophysical determinants of visceral obesity in healthy postmenopausal women. *Int J Obes Relat Metab Disord* 1999;23(8):775–82.

————. The relationship between psychological risk attributes and the metabolic syndrome in healthy women: Antecedent or consequence? *Metabolism* 2002;51(12):1573–77.

Räikkönen, K., K. A. Matthews, L. H. Kuller, et al. Anger, hostility, and visceral adipose tissue in healthy postmenopausal women. *Metabolism* 1999;48(9):1146–51.

Räikkönen, K., K. A. Matthews, and K. Salomon. Hostility predicts metabolic syndrome risk factors in children and adolescents. *Health Psychology* 2003;22(3):279–86.

Rexrode, K. M., A. Pradhan, J. E. Manson, et al. Relationship of total and abdominal adiposity with CRP and IL-6 in women. *Ann Epidemiol* 2003;13(10):674–82.

Rosmond, R. Stress induced disturbances of the HPA axis: A pathway to type 2 diabetes? *Med Sci Monit* 2003;9(2):RA35–RA39.

Rosmond, R., and P. Björntorp. The role of antidepressants in the treatment of abdominal obesity. *Med Hypoth* 2000;54(6):990–94.

Schneider, N., M. Schedlowski, T. H. Schurmeyer, and H. Becker. Stress reduction through music in patients undergoing cerebral angiography. *Neuroradiology* 2001;43(6):472–76.

Smyth, J., M. C. Ockenfels, L. Porter, et al. Stressors and mood measured on a momentary basis are associated with salivary cortisol secretion. *Psychoneuroendocrinology* 1998;23(4):353–70.

Spiegel, K., R. Leproult, and E. Van Cauter. Impact of sleep debt on metabolic and endocrine function. *Lancet* 1999;354(9188):1435–39.

Stockmeier, C. A. Neurobiology of serotonin in depression and suicide. *Ann NY Acad Sci* 1997;836:220–32.

Thakore, J. H., P. J. Richards, R. H. Reznek, et al. Increased intra-abdominal fat deposition in patients with major depressive illness as measured by computed tomography. *Biol Psychiatry* 1997;41:1140–42.

Thomas, S. None of us will ever be the same again: Reactions of American midlife women to 9/11. *Health Care Women Int* 2003;24(10):853–67.

Van Gaal, L. F., M. A. Wauters, and I. H. De Leeuw. Anti-obesity drugs: What does sibutramine offer? An analysis of its potential contribution to obesity treatment. *Exp Clin Endocrinol Diabetes* 1998;106(suppl 2):35–40.

Warnock, J. K., and A. H. Clayton. Chronic episodic disorders in women. *Psychiatr Clin North Am* 2003;26(3):725–40.

Wassertheil-Smoller, S., S. Shumaker, J. Ockene, et al. Depression and cardiovascular sequelae in postmenopausal women. *Arch Intern Med* 2004;164(3):289–98.

Weber-Hamann, B., F. Hentschel, A. Kniest, et al. Hypercortisolemic depression is associated with increased intra-abdominal fat. *Psychosom Med* 2002;64(2):274–77.

Wing, R. R., K. A. Matthews, L. H. Kuller, et al. Waist to hip ratio in middle-aged women: Associations with behavioral and psychosocial factors and with changes in cardiovascular risk factors. *Arterioscler Thromb* 1991;11(5):1250–57.

Chapter 10

Abdel-Hamid, T. K. Exercise and diet in obesity treatment: An integrative system dynamics perspective. *Med Sci Sports Exerc* 2003;35(3):400–13.

Ballor, D. L. Exercise training elevates RMR during moderate but not severe dietary restriction in obese male rats. *J Appl Physiol* 1991;70(5):2303–10.

Ballor, D. L., and E. T. Poehlman. Exercise intensity does not affect depression of resting metabolic rate during severe diet restriction in male Sprague-Dawley rats. *J Nutr* 1993;123(7):1270–76.

———. Exercise-training enhances fat-free mass preservation during diet-induced weight loss: A meta-analytical finding. *Int J Obes Relat Metab Disord* 1994;18(1):35–40.

———. A meta-analysis of the effects of exercise and/or dietary restriction on resting metabolic rate. *Eur J Appl Physiol Occup Physiol* 1995;71(6):535–42.

Ballor, D. L., L. J. Tommerup, D. P. Thomas, et al. Exercise training attenuates diet-induced reduction in metabolic rate. *J Appl Physiol* 1990;68(6):2612–17.

Berry, S. L., W. W. Beatty, and R. C. Klesges. Sensory and social influences on ice cream consumption by males and females in a laboratory setting. *Appetite* 1985;6(1):41–45.

Brownell, K. D. The central role of lifestyle change in long-term weight management. *Clin Cornerstone* 1999;2(3):43–51.

Chandon, P., and B. Wansink. A convenience-salience framework of postpurchase consumption incidence and quantity: When are stockpiled products consumed faster? *J Market Res* 2002;39(3):321–35.

———. Does stockpiling accelerate consumption? A convenience-salience framework of consumption stockpiling. *J Market Res* 2002;39(3):321–35.

Connolly, J., T. Romano, and M. Patruno. Selections from current literature: Effects of dieting and exercise on resting metabolic rate and implications for weight management. *Fam Pract* 1999;16(2):196–201.

Dallman, M. F., N. Pecoraro, S. F. Akana, et al. Chronic stress and obesity: A new view of 'comfort food.' *Proc Natl Acad Sci USA* 2003;100(20):11696–701.

de Castro, J. M. Eating behavior: Lessons from the real world of humans. *Nutrition* 2000;16:800–13.

Donnelly, J. E., N. P. Pronk, D. J. Jacobsen, et al. Effects of a very-low-calorie diet and physical-training regimens on body composition and resting metabolic rate in obese females. *Am J Clin Nutr* 1991;54(1):56–61.

McCargar, I. J. Can diet and exercise really change metabolism? *Medscape General Medicine* 1999;1(1). Internet: www.medscape.com/viewarticle/408808.

Nielsen, S. J., and B. M. Popkin. Patterns and trends in food portion sizes, 1977–1998. *JAMA* 2003;289(4):450–53.

Painter, J. E., B. Wansink, and J. B. Hieggelke. How visibility and convenience influence candy consumption. *Appetite* 2002;38:237–38.

Poehlman, E. T., C. L. Melby, and M. I. Goran. The impact of exercise and diet restriction on daily energy expenditure. *Sports Med* 1991;11(2):78–101.

Roberts, D. C. Quick weight loss: Sorting fad from fact. *Med J Austr* 2001;175:637–40.

Speakman, J. R., and C. Selman. Physical activity and resting metabolic rate. *Proc Nutr Soc* 2003;62(3):621–34.

Wadden, T. A., G. D. Foster, A. J. Stunkard, and A. M. Conill. Effects of weight cycling on the resting energy expenditure and body composition of obese women. *Int J Eat Disord* 1996;19(1):5–12.

Wansink, B., and S. Park. Accessed 2/18/04. At the movies: How external cues and perceived taste impact consumption volume. www.foodpsychologist.com.

Young, L. R., and M. Nestle. The contribution of expanding portion sizes to the US obesity epidemic. *Am J Public Health* 2002;92(2):246–49.

———. Expanding portion sizes in the US marketplace: Implications for nutrition counseling. *J Am Diet Assoc* 2003;103(2):231–34.

Chapter 11

Anderson, J. W., B. M. Johnstone, and M. E. Cook-Newell. Meta-analysis of the effects of soy protein intake on serum lipids. *N Engl J Med* 1995;333:276–82.

Anderson, J. W., K. M. Randles, C. W. Kendall, and D. J. Jenkins. Carbohydrate and fibre recommendations for individuals with diabetes: A quantitative assessment and meta-analysis of the evidence. *J Am Coll Nutr* 2004;23(1):5–17.

Anderson, J. W., B. M. Smith, and N. J. Gustafson. Health benefits and practical aspects of high-fibre diets. *Am J Clin Nutr* 1994;59(5 suppl):1242S– 1247S.

Ascherio, A., and W. C. Willett. Health effects of trans fatty acids. *Am J Clin Nutr* 1997;66(4 suppl):1006S–1010S.

Bazzano, L. A., J. He, L. G. Ogden, et al. Dietary fibre intake and reduced risk of coronary heart disease in US men and women. *Arch Intern Med* 2003;163(16):1897–1904.

Benton, D., and S. Nabb. Carbohydrate, memory, and mood. *Nutr Rev* 2003;61(5):S61–S67.

Bravata, D. M., L. Sanders, J. Huang, et al. Efficacy and safety of low-carbohydrate diets. *JAMA* 2003;289(14):1837–50.

Ciu, H., Y. Yang, L. Bian, and M. He. Effect of food composition of mixed food on glycemic index. Abstract in *Wei Sheng Yan Jiu* (World Journal of Gastroenterology) 1999;28(6):356–58.

Davies, M. J., D. J., Baer, J. T. Judd, et al. Effects of moderate alcohol intake on fasting insulin and glucose concentrations and insulin sensitivity in postmenopausal women. *JAMA* 2002;287(19):2559–62.

Davies, M. J., J. T. Judd, D. J. Baer, et al. Black tea consumption reduces total and LDL cholesterol in mildly hypercholesterolemic adults. *J Nutr* 2003;133(10):3298S–3302S.

Denke, M. A. Metabolic effects of high-protein, low-carbohydrate diets. *Am J Cardiol* 2001;88:59–61.

Despres, J. P., M. C. Pouliot, S. Moorjani, et al. Loss of abdominal fat and metabolic response to exercise training in obese women. *Am J Physiol* 1991;261(2 pt 1):E159–167.

Djousse, L., D. K. Arnett, H. Coon, et al. Fruit and vegetable consumption and LDL cholesterol: The National Heart, Lung, and Blood Institute Family Heart Study. *Am J Clin Nutr* 2004;79(2):213–17.

Ford, E. S., and A. H. Mokdad. Fruit and vegetable consumption and diabetes mellitus incidence among U.S. adults. *Prev Med* 2001;32(1):33–39.

Foster, G. D., H. R. Wyatt, J. O. Hill, et al. A randomized trial of a low-carbohydrate diet for obesity. *N Engl J Med* 2003;348(21):2082–90.

Franz, M. J. The answer to weight loss is easy – doing it is hard! *Clinical Diabetes* 2001;19:105–08.

Franz, M. J., J. P. Bantle, C. A. Beebe, et al. Nutrition principles and recommendations in diabetes. *Diabetes Care* 2004;27(suppl 1):S36–S46.

Gago-Dominguez, M, J. M. Yuan, C. L. Sun, et al. Opposing effects of dietary n-3 and n-6 fatty acids on mammary carcinogenesis: The Singapore Chinese Health Study. *Br J Cancer* 2003;89(9):1686–92.

Gardner, C. D., K. A. Newell, R. Cherin, and W. L. Haskell. The effect of soy protein with or without isoflavones relative to milk protein on plasma lipids in hypercholesterolemic postmenopausal women. *Am J Clin Nutr* 2001;73:728–35.

Golay, A., A. F. Allaz, Y. Morel, et al. Similar weight loss with low- or high-carbohydrate diets. *Am J Clin Nutr* 1996;63(2):174–78.

Goodman-Gruen, D., and D. Kritz-Silverstein. Usual dietary isoflavone intake and body composition in postmenopausal women. *Menopause* 2003;10(5): 427–32.

Hasler, C. M. The cardiovascular effects of soy products. *J Cardiovasc Nurs* 2002;16(4):50–63.

Hays, N. P., R. D. Starling, X. Liu, et al. Effects of an ad libitum low-fat, high-carbohydrate diet on body weight, body composition, and fat distribution in older men and women. *Arch Intern Med* 2004;164:210–17.

Horton, T. J., H. Drougas, A. Brachey, et al. Fat and carbohydrate overfeeding in humans: Different effects on energy storage. *Am J Clin Nutr* 1995;62(1):19–29.

Hu, F. B., J. E. Manson, and W. C. Willett. Types of dietary fat and risk of coronary heart disease: A critical review. *J Am Coll Nutr* 2001;20(1):5–19.

Hu, F. B., M. J. Stampfer, J. E. Manson, et al. Frequent nut consumption and risk of coronary heart disease in women: Prospective cohort study. *BMJ* 1998;317:1341–1345.

Jacobs, E. J., C. J. Connell, A. Chao, et al. Multivitamin use and colorectal cancer incidence in a US cohort: Does timing matter? *Am J Epidemiol* 2003;158(7):621–28.

Jenkins, D. J., C. W. Kendall, C. J. Jackson, et al. Effects of high- and low-isoflavone soyfoods on blood lipids, oxidized LDL, homocysteine, and blood pressure in hyperlipidemic men and women. *Am J Clin Nutr* 2002;76(2):365–72.

Jiang, R., J. E. Manson, M. J. Stampfer, et al. Nut and peanut butter consumption and risk of type 2 diabetes in women. *JAMA* 2002;288(20):2554–60.

Jones, P. R. M., and D. A. Edwards. Areas of fat loss in overweight young females following an 8-week period of energy intake reduction. *Ann Human Biol* 1999;26(2):151–62.

Keith, R. E., K. A. O'Keeffe, D. L. Blessing, and G. D. Wilson. Alterations in dietary carbohydrate, protein, and fat intake and mood state in trained female cyclists. *Med Sci Sports Exerc* 1991;23(2):212–16.

Landers, P., M. M. Wolfe, S. Glore, et al. Effect of weight loss plans on body composition and diet duration. *J Okla State Med Assoc* 2002;95(5):329–31.

Lichtenstein, A. H. Got soy? *Am J Clin Nutr* 2001;73:667–68.

Liu, S., J. E. Manson, I.-M. Lee, et al. Fruit and vegetable intake and risk of cardiovascular disease: The Women's Health Study. *Am J Clin Nutr* 2000;72:922–28.

Liu, S., J. E. Manson, M. J. Stampfer, et al. A prospective study of whole-grain intake and risk of type 2 diabetes mellitus in US women. *Am J Public Health* 2000;90(9):1409–15.

Liu, S., M. J. Stampfer, F. B. Hu, et al. Whole-grain consumption and risk of coronary heart disease: Results from the Nurses' Health Study. *Am J Clin Nutr* 1999;70(3):412–19.

Ludwig, D. S. The glycemic index: Physiological mechanisms relating to obesity, diabetes, and cardiovascular disease. *JAMA* 2002;287(18):2414–23.

Mann, J. I. Can dietary intervention produce long-term reduction in insulin resistance? *Br J Nutr* 2000;83(suppl 1):S169–S172.

Markus, R., G. Panhuysen, A. Tuiten, and H. Koppeschaar. Effects of food on cortisol and mood in vulnerable subjects under controllable and uncontrollable stress. *Physiol Behav* 2000;70:333–42.

Marshall, J. A., R. F. Hamman, and J. Baxter. High-fat, low-carbohydrate diet and the etiology of non-insulin-dependent diabetes mellitus: The San Luis Valley Diabetes Study. *Am J Epidemiol* 1991;134(6):590–603.

Marshall, J. A., S. Hoag, S. Shetterly, and R. F. Hamman. Dietary fat predicts conversion from impaired glucose tolerance to NIDDM: The San Luis Valley Diabetes Study. *Diabetes Care* 1994;17(1):50–56.

McKeown, N. M., J. B. Miegs, S. Liu, et al. Carbohydrate nutrition, insulin resistance, and the prevalence of the metabolic syndrome in the Framingham Offspring Cohort. *Diabetes Care* 2004;27(2):538–46.

Meyer, K. A., L. H. Kushi, D. R. Jacobs, et al. Carbohydrates, dietary fibre, and incident type 2 diabetes in older women. *Am J Clin Nutr* 2000;71(4):921–30.

Newby, P. K., D. Muller, J. Hallfrisch, et al. Dietary patterns and changes in body mass index and waist circumference in adults. *Am J Clin Nutr* 2003;77(6):1417–25.

Nicklas, B. J., K. E. Dennis, D. M. Berman, et al. Lifestyle intervention of hypocaloric dieting and walking reduces abdominal obesity and improves coronary heart disease risk factors in obese, postmenopausal, African-American and Caucasian women. *J Gerontol A Biol Sci Med Sci* 2003;58(2):181–89.

Park, H. S., and K. U. Lee. Postmenopausal women lose less visceral adipose tissue during a weight reduction program. *Menopause* 2003;10(3):222–27.

Pelkman, C. L., V. K. Fishell, D. H. Maddox, et al. Effects of moderate-fat (from monounsaturated fat) and low-fat weight loss diets on the serum lipid profile in overweight and obese men and women. *Am J Clin Nutr* 2004;79(2):204–12.

Pi-Sunyer, F. X. Glycemic index and disease. *Am J Clin Nutr* 2002;76(1):290S–298S.

Pirozzo, S., C. Summerbell, C. Cameron, and P. Glasziou. Should we recommend low-fat diets for obesity? *Obes Rev* 2003;4:83–90.

Riccardi, G., G. Clement, and R. Giacco. Glycemic index of local foods and diets: The Mediterranean experience. *Nutr Rev* 2003;61(5):S56–S60.

Rimm, E. B., W. C. Willett, F. B. Hu, et al. Folate and vitamin B6 from diet and supplements in relation to risk of coronary heart disease among women. *JAMA* 1998;279(5):359–64.

Rodríguez-Morán, M., F. Guerrero-Romero, and G. Lazcano-Burciaga. Lipid-

and glucose-lowering efficacy of Plantago psyllium in type 2 diabetes. *J Diabetes Complications* 1998;12(5):273–8.

Ryan, M., D. McInerney, D. Owens, et al. Diabetes and the Mediterranean diet: A beneficial effect of oleic acid on insulin sensitivity, adipocyte glucose transport and endothelium-dependent vasoreactivity. *J Med* 2000;93: 85–91.

Ryan, A. S., B. J. Nicklas, D. M. Berman, and K. E. Dennis. Dietary restriction and walking reduce fat deposition in the midthigh in obese older women. *Am J Clin Nutr* 2000;72:708–13.

Sabaté, J. Nut consumption and body weight. *Am J Clin Nutr* 2003;78(3 suppl):647S–650S.

Sabaté, J., G. E. Fraser, K. Burke, et al. Effects of walnuts on serum lipid levels and blood pressure in normal men. *N Engl J Med* 1993;328(9):603–07.

Salmerón, J., H. B. Hu, J. E. Manson, et al. Dietary fat intake and risk of type 2 diabetes in women. *Am J Clin Nutr* 2001;73:1019–26.

Salmerón, J., J. E. Manson, M. J. Stampfer, et al. Dietary fibre, glycemic load, and risk of non-insulin-dependent diabetes mellitus in women. *JAMA* 1997;277(6):472–77.

Saris, W. H. M. Glycemic carbohydrate and body weight regulation. *Nutr Rev* 2003;61(5):S10–S16.

Schweiger, U., R. Laessle, S. Kittl, et al. Macronutrient intake, plasma large neutral amino acids and mood during weight-reducing diets. *J Neural Transm* 1986;67(1–2):77–86.

Smith, S. R., and J. J. Zachwieja. Visceral adipose tissue: A critical review of intervention strategies. *Int J Obes Relat Metab Disord* 1999;23(4):329–35.

Solomon, C. G., F. B. Hu, M. J. Stampfer, et al. Moderate alcohol consumption and risk of coronary heart disease among women with type 2 diabetes mellitus. *Circulation* 2000;102:494–99.

Stubbs, R. J., P. Ritz, W. A. Coward, and A. M. Prentice. Covert manipulation of the ratio of dietary fat to carbohydrate and energy density: Effect on food intake and energy balance in free-living men eating ad libitum. *Am J Clin Nutr* 1995;62(2):330–37.

Tian, W. X., L. C. Li, X. D. Wu, and C. C. Che. Weight reduction by Chinese medicinal herbs may be related to inhibition of fatty acid synthase. *Life Sci* 2004;74(19):2389–99.

Toubro, S., and A. Astrup. Randomised comparison of diets for maintaining obese subjects' weight after major weight loss: Ad lib, low fat, high carbohydrate diet v. fixed energy intake. *BMJ* 1997;314:29–34.

Tuomilehto, J., G. Hu, S. Bidel, et al. Coffee consumption and risk of type 2 diabetes mellitus among middle-aged Finnish men and women. *JAMA* 2004;291(10):1213–19.

Wabitsch, M., H. Hauner, A. Bockmann, et al. The relationship between body fat distribution and weight loss in obese adolescent girls. *Int J Obes Relat Metab Disord* 1992;16(11):905–11.

Wannamethee, S. C., C. A. Camargo Jr., J. E. Manson, et al. Alcohol drinking patterns and risk of type 2 diabetes mellitus among younger women. *Arch Intern Med* 2003;163(11):1329–36.

Wansink, B., S. B. Park, S. Sonka, and M. Morganosky. Ingredient disclosure and product acceptance: How soy labeling influences preference and taste. *Intl Food Agribusinss Manag Rev* 2000;3:85–94.

Willett, W., J. Manson, and S. Liu. Glycemic index, glycemic load, and risk of type 2 diabetes. *Am J Clin Nutr* 2002;76(1):274S–280S.

Wolever, T. M., D. J. Jenkins, S. Mueller, et al. Method of administration influences the serum cholesterol-lowering effect of psyllium. *Am J Clin Nutr* 1994;59(5):1055–59.

Wollin, S. K., and P. J. H. Jones. Alcohol, red wine and cardiovascular disease. *J Nutr* 2001;131:1401–04.

Wu, C. H., F. H. Lu, C. S. Chang, et al. Relationship among habitual tea consumption, per cent body fat, and body fat distribution. *Obes Res* 2003;11(9):1088–95.

Chapter 12

Albertazzi, P., and D. W. Purdie. The nature and utility of the phytooestrogens: A review of the evidence. *Maturitas* 2002;42:173–85.

Arjmandi, B. H., D. A. Khalil, B. J. Smith, et al. Soy protein has a greater effect on bone in postmenopausal women not on hormone replacement therapy, as evidenced by reducing bone resorption and urinary calcium excretion. *J Clin Endocrinol Metab* 2003;88(3):1048–54.

Camara-Martos, F., and M. A. Amaro-Lopez. Influence of dietary factors on calcium bioavailability: A brief review. *Biol Trace Elem Res* 2002;89(1):43–52.

Chen, Y. M., S. C. Ho, S. S. Lam, et al. Soy isoflavones have a favorable effect on bone loss in Chinese postmenopausal women with lower bone mass: A double-blind, randomized, controlled trial. *J Clin Endocrinol Metab* 2003;88(10):4740–47.

Freese, J., and S. Meland. Seven tenths incorrect: Heterogeneity and change in the waist-to-hip ratios of *Playboy* centerfold models and Miss America Pageant winners. *J Sex Res* 2002;39(2):133–38.

Guillen, E. O., and S. I. Barr. Nutrition, dieting, and fitness messages in a magazine for adolescent women, 1970–1990. *J Adolesc Health* 1994;15(6):464–72.

Gupta, M. A., S. K. Chaturvedi, P. C. Chandarana, and A. M. Johnson. Weight-related body image concerns among 18–24-year-old women in Canada and India: An empirical comparative study. *J Psychosom Res* 2001;50:193–98.

Hays, N. P., R. D. Starling, X. Liu, et al. Effects of an ad libitum low-fat, high-carbohydrate diet on body weight, body composition, and fat distribution in older men and women. *Arch Intern Med* 2004;164:210–17.

Ho, S. C., J. Woo, S. Lam, et al. Soy protein consumption and bone mass in early postmenopausal Chinese women. *Osteoporos Int* 2003;14(10):835–42.

Hoffman, J. M., and K. D. Brownell. Sex differences in the relationship of body fat distribution with psychosocial variables. *Int J Eat Disord* 1997;22:139–45.

Ishida, H., H. Takahashi, H. Suzuki, et al. Interrelationship of some selected nutritional parameters relevant to taste for salt in a group of college-aged women. *J Nutr Sci Vitaminol* (Tokyo) 1985;31(6):585–98.

Lewis, C. M. Dissatisfaction among women with 'thunder thighs' undergoing closed aspirative lipoplasty. *Aesthetic Plast Surg* 1987;11(3):187–91.

L'Hermitte, F., A. Behar, J. Paries, et al. Impairment of lymphatic function in women with gynoid adiposity and swelling syndrome. *Metabolism* 2003;52(7):805–09.

Lindeman, A. K. Quest for ideal weight: Costs and consequences. *Med Sci Sports Exerc* 1999;31(8):1135–40.

Macdonald, H. M., S. A. New, M. H. Golden, et al. Nutritional associations with bone loss during the menopausal transition: Evidence of a beneficial effect of calcium, alcohol, and fruit and vegetable nutrients and of a detrimental effect of fatty acids. *Am J Clin Nutr* 2004;79(1):155–65.

McCarty, M. F. A paradox resolved: The postprandial model of insulin resistance explains why gynoid adiposity appears to be protective. *Med Hypoth* 2003;61(2):173–76.

Messina, M. J. Soy foods and soybean isoflavones and menopausal health. *Nutr Clin Care* 2002;5(6):272–82.

Mojet, J., E. Christ-Hazelhop, and J. Heidema. Taste perception with age:

Generic or specific losses in threshold sensitivity to the five basic tastes? *Chem Senses* 2001;26(7):845–60.

Moore, D. C. Body image and eating behavior in adolescents. *J Am Coll Nutr* 1993;12(5):505–10.

Morris, A., T. Cooper, and P. J. Cooper. The changing shape of female fashion models. *Int J Eating Disord* 1989;8:593–96.

Nagata, C., N. Takatsuka, N. Kawakami, and H. Shimizu. Soy product intake and hot flashes in Japanese women: Results from a community-based prospective study. *Am J Epidemiol* 2001;153(8):790–93.

Osada, K., M. Komai, B. P. Bryant, et al. Age related decreases in neural sensitivity to NaCl in SHR-SP. *J Vet Med Sci* 2003;65(3):313–17.

Philp, H. A. Hot flashes – a review of the literature on alternative and complementary treatment approaches. *Altern Med Rev* 2003;8(3):284–302.

Poppitt, S. D., G. F. Keogh, A. M. Prentice, et al. Long-term effects of ad libitum low-fat, high-carbohydrate diets on body weight and serum lipids in overweight subjects with metabolic syndrome. *Am J Clin Nutr* 2002;75:11–20.

Shapses, S. A., S. Heshka, and S. B. Heymsfield. Effect of calcium supplementation on weight and fat loss in women. *J Clin Endocrinol Metab* 2004;89(2):632–37.

Shimatani, Y., S. Nikles, K. Najafi, and R. M. Bradley. Long-term recordings from afferent taste fibers. *Physiol Behav* 2003;80(2–3):309–15.

Summers, L. K. M., B. A. Fielding, H. A. Bradshaw, et al. Substituting dietary saturated fat with polyunsaturated fat changes abdominal fat distribution and improves insulin sensitivity. *Diabetologia* 2002;45(3):369–77.

Tucker, K. L., H. Chen, M. T. Hannan, et al. Bone mineral density and dietary patterns in older adults: The Framingham Osteoporosis study. *Am J Clin Nutr* 2002;76(1):245–52.

Tucker, K. L., M. T. Hannan, H. Chen, et al. Potassium, magnesium, and fruit and vegetable intakes are associated with greater bone mineral density in elderly men and women. *Am J Clin Nutr* 1999;69:727–36.

Voracek, M., and M. L. Fisher. Shapely centrefolds? Temporal change in body measures: Trend analysis. *BMJ* 2002;325:1447–48.

Weststrate, J. A., J. Dekker, M. Stoel, et al. Resting energy expenditure in women: Impact of obesity and body-fat distribution. *Metabolism* 1990;39(1):11–17.

Wiseman, C. V., J. J. Gray, J. E. Mosimann, and A. H. Aherns. Cultural expectations of thinness in women: An update. *Int J Eating Disord* 1992;11:85–89.

Zemel, M. B. Role of dietary calcium and dairy products in modulating adiposity. *Lipids* 2003;38(2):139–46.

Chapter 13

Babyak, M., J. A. Blumenthal, S. Herman, et al. Exercise treatment for major depression: Maintenance of therapeutic benefit at 10 months. *Psychosom Med* 2000;62(5):633–38.

Barnes, D. E., K. Yaffe, W. A. Satariano, and I. B. Tager. A longitudeinal study of cardiorespiratory fitness and cognitive function in healthy older adults. *J Am Geriatr Soc* 2003;51(4):459–65.

Bauldoff, G. S., L. A. Hoffman, T. G. Zullo, and F. C. Sciurba. Exercise maintenance following pulmonary rehabilitation: Effect of distractive stimuli. *Chest* 2002;122(3):948–54.

Bemben, D. A., N. L. Fetters, M. G. Bemben, et al. Musculoskeletal responses to high- and low-intensity resistance training in early postmenopausal women. *Med Sci Sports Exerc* 2000;32(11):1949–57.

Blundell, J. E., and N. A. King. Effects of exercise on appetite control: Loose coupling between energy expenditure and energy intake. *Int J Obes Relat Metab Disord* 1998;22(suppl 2):S22–S29.

Bond Brill, J., A. C. Perry, L. Parker, et al. Dose-response effect of walking exercise on weight loss. How much is enough? *Int J Obes Relat Metab Disord* 2002;26(11):1484–93.

Chakravarthy, M. V., M. J. Joyner, and F. W. Booth. An obligation for primary care physicians to prescribe physical activity to sedentary patients to reduce the risk of chronic health conditions. *Mayo Clin Proc* 2002;77:165–73.

Cuff, D. J., G. S. Meneilly, A. Martin, et al. Effective exercise modality to reduce insulin resistance in women with type 2 diabetes. *Diabetes Care* 2003;26:2977–82.

Cussler, E. C., T. G. Lohman, S. B. Going, et al. Weight lifted in strength training predicts bone change in postmenopausal women. *Med Sci Sports Exerc* 2003;35:10–17.

Damush, T. M., and J. G. Damush Jr. The effects of strength training on strength and health-related quality of life in older adult women. *Gerontologist* 1999;39(6):705–10.

De Bourdeaudhuij, I., G. Crombez, B. Deforche, et al. Effects of distraction on treadmill running time in severely obese children and adolescents. *Int J Obes Relat Metab Disord* 2002;26(8):1023–29.

Donnelly, J. E., J. O. Hill, D. J. Jacobsen, et al. Effects of a 16-month randomized controlled exercise trial on body weight and composition in young, overweight men and women: The Midwest Exercise Trial. *Arch Intern Med* 2003;163:1343–50.

Douchi, T., S. Yamamoto, T. Oki, et al. The effects of physical exercise on body fat distribution and bone mineral density in postmenopausal women. *Maturitas* 2000;35:25–30.

Ekkekakis, P., E. E. Hall, and S. J. Petruzzello. Practical markers of the transition from aerobic to anaerobic metabolism during exercise: Rationale and a case for affect-based exercise prescription. *Prev Med* 2004;38(2):149–59.

Evans, E. M., R. E. Van Pelt, E. F. Binder, et al. Effects of HRT and exercise training on insulin action, glucose tolerance, and body composition in older women. *J Appl Physiol* 2001;90:2033–40.

Folland, J. P., C. S. Irish, J. C. Roberts, et al. Fatigue is not a necessary stimulus for strength gains during resistance training. *Br J Sports Med* 2002;36(5):370–73.

Gregg, E. W., J. A. Cauley, K. Stone, et al. Relationship of changes in physical activity and mortality among older women. *JAMA* 2003;289(18):2379–86.

Hu, F. B. R. J. Sigal, J. W. Rich-Edwards, et al. Walking compared with vigorous physical activity and risk of type 2 diabetes in women: A prospective study. *JAMA* 1999;282(15):1433–39.

Hu, F. B., M. J. Stampfer, G. A. Colditz, et al. Physical activity and risk of stroke in women. *JAMA* 2000;283(22):2961–67.

Hu, F. B., M. J. Stampfer, C. Solomon, et al. Physical activity and risk of cardiovascular events in diabetic women. *Ann Intern Med* 2001;134(2):96–105.

Hurley, B. F., and S. M. Roth. Strength training in the elderly: Effects on risk factors for age-related diseases. *Sports Med* 2000;30(4):249–68.

Irwin, M. L., Y. Yasui, C. M. Ulrich, et al. Effect of exercise on total and intra-abdominal body fat in postmenopausal women: A randomized controlled trial. *JAMA* 2003;289(3):323–30.

Layne, J. E., and M. E. Nelson. The effects of progressive resistance training on bone density: A review. *Med Sci Sports Exerc* 1999;31(1):25–30.

Manson, J. E., F. B. Hu, J. W. Rich-Edwards, et al. A prospective study of walking as compared with vigorous exercise in the prevention of coronary heart disease in women. *N Engl J Med* 1999;341(9):650–58.

Manson, J. E., D. M. Nathan, A. S. Krolewski, et al. A prospective study of exercise and incidence of diabetes among US male physicians. *JAMA* 1992;268(1):63–67.

Mayo, M. J., J. R. Grantham, and B. Govindasamy. Exercise-induced weight loss preferentially reduces abdominal fat. *Med Sci Sports Exerc* 2003;35(2):207–13.

McTiernan, A., C. Kooperberg, E. White, et al. Recreational physical activity and the risk of breast cancer in postmenopausal women: The Women's Health Initiative cohort study. *JAMA* 2003;290(10):1331–36.

Meston, C. M., and B. B. Gorzalka. Differential effects of sympathetic activation on sexual arousal in sexually dysfunctional and functional women. *J Abnorm Psychol* 1996;105(4):582–91.

Nelson, M. E., M. A. Fiatarone, C. M. Morganti, et al. Effects of high-intensity strength training on multiple risk factors for osteoporotic fractures: A randomized controlled trial. *JAMA* 1994;272(24):1909–14.

North American Menopause Society. Treatment of menopause-associated vasomotor symptoms: Position statement of The North American Menopause Society. *Menopause* 2004;11(1):11–33.

Park, S. K., J. H. Park, Y.-C. Kwon, et al. The effect of combined aerobic and resistance exercise training on abdominal fat in obese middle-aged women. *J Physiol Anthropol* 2003;22(3):129–35.

Poulton, R., J. Trevena, A. I. Reedeer, and R. Richaards. Physical health correlates of overprediction of physical discomfort during exercise. *Behav Res Therapy* 2002;40(4):401–14.

Rogers, M. E., H. S. Sherwood, N. L. Rogers, and R. M. Bohlken. Effects of dumbbell and elastic band training on physical function in older inner-city African-American women. *Women Health* 2002;36(4):33–41.

Samaras, K., P. J. Kelly, M. N. Chiano, et al. Genetic and environmental influences on total-body and central abdominal fat: The effect of physical activity in female twins. *Ann Intern Med* 1999;130:873–82.

Saris, W. H. M., S. N. Blair, M. A. van Baak, et al. How much physical activity is enough to prevent unhealthy weight gain? Outcome of the IASO 1st Stock Conference and Consensus Statement. *Obesity Rev* 2003;4:101–114.

Singh, R. B., V. Rastogi, S. S. Rastogi, et al. Effect of diet and moderate exercise on central obesity and associated disturbances, myocardial infarction and mortality in patients with and without coronary artery disease. *J Am Coll Nutr* 1996;15(6):592–601.

Slentz, C. A., B. D. Duscha, J. L. Johnson, et al. Effects of the amount of exercise on body weight, body composition, and measures of central obesity: STRRIDE – a randomized controlled study. *Arch Intern Med* 2004;164:31–39.

Index

waist circumference reduction and,
29–30
Lowell, Amy, 254
Low-fat snacks, 272
Lucozade, 267
Lunch, food choices for, 243–245,
280–282

M

Magnetic resonance imaging (MRI), of
breast, 129
Mammograms, 129
Meat substitutes, 232–233
Medications
diabetes effects of, 90–92
and diabetes prevention, 93–95
and HPA axis reactivity, 170–171
for inflammation and cardiovascular
disease, 110–114
and osteoporosis, 145–146
Menopause
body shape and, 43–44
hormones during, 60–63
Menstrual cycle, hormones during,
50–51
Metabolic syndrome, 79–97
metabolism in, 85–86
prevention of, 92–95
Metabolism, 38, 82–87, 186–188
Metformin, 93–94
Metoprolol, for high blood pressure,
111
Micronor, 56
Microval, 56
Midmeal break, 205
Midmorning snack, food choices for,
241–243, 278–280
Mind-body connection, 155–157
Moderate foods, 274

Moduretic, for high blood pressure,
111, 113
Monounsaturated fats, 224, 269
MRI, of breast, 129
Multivitamins, 239–240, 277–278
Muscle mass
and bone density, 139–140
and metabolism, 186–187
Myocardial infarction, 102

N

Neurons, 153
Neurotransmitters, 153
Niacin, for high blood fats, 112
Norelgestromin with ethinyl oestradiol,
55–56
Norethindrone, 56
Nutrition, 179–209
basics of, 183–186
reality check on, 180–183
Nuts, 227–228
Nuvelle, 72

O

Obesity
and bone density, 138
and breast cancer, 122–123
in children, 38–39
definitions of, 19–20
Oestradiol, 61
Oestrogen, 8–9, 49–51
menopause and, 60–61
Oestrone, 61
Olanzapine, 92
Omega-3 fatty acids, 225, 269
Omega-6 fatty acids, 225, 269–270
Oral contraceptives, 53–58
contraindications to, 54–55

Q

Quetiapine, 92
Quinoa, 250

R

Ramipril, for high blood pressure, 110
Reasons for not exercising, 288–289
  dealing with, 296–301
Recipes, experimenting with, 207, 247
Red clover, 73
Reductil, and HPA axis reactivity,
  171
Remifemin, 73–74
Resistance exercise, 294, 305–307
  for osteoporosis prevention, 143
  programme of, 308–320
Reverse Crunch, 320, *320*
Risendronate, for osteoporosis, 145
Risotto, 284
Risperdal (risperidone), 92
Rosiglitazone, 94

S

Safety, and exercise, 300–301
Salt, 265–267, 274
Satisfaction, clues to, 195–196
Saturated fats, 224, 269
Sautéeing, 247–248
Seasonale, 54
Selective estrogen receptor modulators
  (SERMs), cautions with, 145–146
Self-care, 117
Seroquel, 92
Seroxat, 75
Serving sizes, 197–199
Shoulder exercises, 309, *309,* 310,
  310

Sibutramine, and HPA axis reactivity,
  171
Simvastatin, for high blood fats, 112
Sleep
  and cancer prevention, 130
  and diabetes prevention, 96
Slim foods, 273
Smoking cessation
  for cancer prevention, 129
  and diabetes prevention, 92–93
  for inflammation and cardiovascular
    disease, 109
  for osteoporosis prevention, 142
Snack mix, 280
Snacks
  afternoon, 247, 282
  evening, 251, 286
  food choices for, 241–243, 278–280
  low-carb, 243
  low-fat, 272
  visibility of, 199
Society, and health, 190–191
Sodium, 265–267, 274
Soluble fibre, 222
Soya butter, 233
Soya foods, 74–75, 229–233,
    263–265, 274
  adding to diet, 232–233
  health benefits of, 231–232
  psychology of, 230–231
Soya milk, 233
Sports drinks, 267
Statin medications, for high blood fats,
  112
Steroids, 90–91
  and osteoporosis, 145
Stomach exercises, 308, *308,* 320, *320*
Strength training. *See* resistance
  exercise
Stress, 153–175